ALSO BY EMILY OSTER

*Expecting Better: Why the Conventional Pregnancy Wisdom
Is Wrong—and What You Really Need to Know*

EMILY OSTER is a professor of economics at Brown University and the author of *Expecting Better*. She spoke at the 2007 TED conference and has been featured in *The New York Times*, the *Wall Street Journal*, *Forbes* and *Esquire*. Oster is married to economist Jesse Shapiro and is also the daughter of two economists. She has two children.

'Emily Oster is the non-judgemental girlfriend holding our hand and guiding us through pregnancy and motherhood. She has done the work to get us the hard facts in a soft, understandable way.' Amy Schumer

'Shows that in the hectic haze of parenthood an economist's perspective can prove surprisingly clarifying.' *Economist*

'She has crunched all the statistics on breastfeeding, potty training, working mothers and playgroups and discovered there is no optimal set of choices that will produce the perfect child. Most parents say they want happy, well-adjusted, robust kids and there are myriad ways to achieve those results. She's right.' *The Times*

'It couldn't be more relevant ... steers clear of recommendations and cast-iron guarantees, instead promising to arm parents with information to make the decisions that are right for them' *Daily Telegraph*

'A huge relief from the scare stories ... *Cribsheet* is not another call for the end of helicopter parenting or snowplow parenting or whatever kind of parenting is lighting up social media today, and it's not a call to overthrow medical wisdom; it's a call for parenting with context, and it's freeing.' *Washington Post*

'Both refreshing and useful. With so many parenting theories driving us all a bit batty, this is the type of book that we need to help calm things down.' *L.A. Times*

'The guilt-free, data-driven guide to parenting ... uses science and stats to cut through the confusion of raising a family ... Smart, relatable, and funny.' *Bloomberg*

Cribsheet

*A Data-Driven Guide to Better,
More Relaxed Parenting,
from Birth to Preschool*

EMILY OSTER

SOUVENIR
PRESS

This paperback edition published in 2020

First published in Great Britain in 2019 by Souvenir Press,
an imprint of Profile Books Ltd
29 Cloth Fair
London EC1A 7JQ
www.profilebooks.com

First published in the USA by Penguin Press, an imprint of Penguin Random House LLC

ISBN 978 1 78816 449 8
eISBN 978 1 78283 655 1
Audio ISBN: 978 1 78283 659 9

Printed and bound in Great Britain by CPI Group (UK) Ltd, Croydon CR0 4YY

To Penelope and Finn

CONTENTS

Introduction   *xiii*

PART ONE

In the Beginning

1. The First Three Days   *5*

2. Wait, You Want Me to Take It Home?   *28*

3. Trust Me, Take the Mesh Underwear   *41*

PART TWO

The First Year

4. Breast Is Best? Breast Is Better? Breast Is About the Same?   *65*

5. Breastfeeding: A How-To Guide   *88*

6. Sleep Position and Location   *111*

7. Organize Your Baby   *128*

8. Vaccination: Yes, Please   *135*

9. Stay-at-Home Mom? Stay-at-Work Mom? *148*

10. Who Should Take Care of the Baby? *159*

11. Sleep Training *171*

12. Beyond the Boobs: Introducing Solid Food *188*

PART THREE

From Baby to Toddler

13. Early Walking, Late Walking: Physical Milestones *209*

14. Baby Einstein vs. the TV Habit *217*

15. Slow Talking, Fast Talking: Language Development *228*

16. Potty Training: Stickers vs. M&M's *238*

17. Toddler Discipline *250*

18. Education *259*

PART FOUR

The Home Front

19. Internal Politics *273*

20. Expansions *282*

21. Growing Up and Letting Go *289*

Acknowledgments *293*
Appendix: Further Reading *295*
Notes *297*
Index *313*

Cribsheet

INTRODUCTION

As infants, both my children loved to be swaddled—wrapped up tightly in blankets to sleep. Our blanket of choice was something called the Miracle Blanket, which involved a complicated wrapping procedure that only Houdini himself could have escaped. We had about nine of these blankets, since we feared we would run out and have to use a swaddle covered in poop.

Swaddling is great, and it *can* help your infant sleep. But there is a downside: you can't use it forever. At some point, your kid will get too big and you'll have to stop. Now, a first-time parent might not assume that this is a problem, but breaking the swaddle habit is no easy task.

With our daughter, Penelope (kid number one), breaking the swaddle led to worse sleep habits, followed by a long reliance on a product called the Rock 'n Play Sleeper, which I still have nightmares about. Other parents have told me stories of seeking secret online sources for larger-size swaddles. There *are* women on Etsy who will create a swaddle blanket for your eighteen-month-old. Please note: Just because there is a secret market for something on Etsy doesn't necessarily mean it's a good idea.

One of the features of having a second child is you can have a do-over on all your perceived mistakes. As an "experienced parent," you can make sure that anything you look back on with regret you'll fix on this round.

At least, that's what I thought. Breaking the swaddle was at the top of my list. I was going to do it right this time.

As Finn (kid number two) approached four or five months old, I made a plan. First, for a few days I'd swaddle Finn as usual, but leave one arm uncovered. Then, a few days later, after he adjusted to that, I'd take the other arm out. Then I'd uncover his legs. Finally, I'd dispense with the whole swaddle. The internet assured me that this way we'd lose the swaddle without also losing any (hard-won) sleeping skills.

I was ready to start. I put a date on the calendar and informed my husband, Jesse.

Then, one extremely hot day shortly before the assigned start date, the power went out, and with it the air conditioning. Finn's room was 95 degrees. It was approaching bedtime. I panicked. When fully deployed, the swaddle blanket was many layers of fabric. Finn would roast.

Should I keep him awake in the hopes the power would come back on? It could be days. Should I just swaddle him and figure he'd be hot? This seemed irresponsible and also kind of mean. Should I just hold him while he slept and not put him in the crib at all until it cooled down? This was also very hot, and experience suggested he wouldn't sleep for long in my arms.

My best-laid plans set aside, I put him to bed in a diaper and onesie. No swaddle. I explained it to him as I nursed him to sleep, drenched in sweat.

"Finn, I'm sorry, but it's so hot out! We can't use the swaddle. But don't worry, you can still sleep. I know you can do it! Now you'll be able to suck on your fingers! Won't that be nice?"

With a big smile, I put him in his crib, unswaddled, and left the room. I prepared for the worst. Penelope would have screamed bloody murder. Finn, though, just made a few surprised noises and fell asleep.

Obviously, an hour later the power came back on. By then Finn was sleeping. I asked Jesse if I should go in and swaddle him now. Jesse told me I was nuts, and collected all the Miracle Blankets for the charity bin.

As I lay in bed that night, I wondered if Finn would sleep worse now, if

I should go dig the blankets out of the bin and wrap him in one. I was tempted to jump on the computer and read stories of swaddle-induced sleep regression, or lack thereof. In the end, I was too hot to follow through, and our swaddle days were over.

As a parent, you want nothing more than to do the right thing for your children, to make the best choices for them. At the same time, it can be impossible to know what those best choices are. Things crop up that you never thought about—even with a second kid, probably even with a fifth kid. The world, and your child, surprise you all the time. It is hard not to second-guess yourself, even on the small things.

The swaddle breaking was, of course, a tiny incident. But it illustrates what will be one of the great themes of your parenting life: you have way less control than you think you do. You might ask why, if I know this to be true, have I written a guide to parenting in the early years? The answer is that you do have choices, even if not control, and these choices are important. The problem is that the atmosphere around parenting rarely frames these choices in a way that gives parents autonomy.

We can do better, and data and economics, surprisingly, can help. My goal with this book is to take some of the stress out of the early years by arming you with good information and a method for making the best decisions for your family.

I also hope *Cribsheet* will offer a basic, data-derived map of the big issues that come up in the first three years of being a parent. I found that hard to come by in my own experience.

Most of us are parenting later than our parents did; we've been functional adults a lot longer than any previous generation of new parents. That's not just a neat demographic fact. It means we're used to autonomy, and thanks to technology, we are used to having pretty much limitless information in our decision-making.

We'd like to approach parenting the same way, but the sheer number of decisions causes information overload. Especially early on, every day seems to have another challenge, and when you look for advice, everyone says something different. And, frankly, they all seem like experts relative to you. It's daunting even before you factor in your depleted postpartum state and the tiny new resident of your home who won't latch onto your breast, sleep, or stop screaming. Take a deep breath.

There are many big decisions: Should you breastfeed? Should you sleep train, and with what method? What about allergies? Some people say avoid peanuts, others say give them to your child as soon as possible—which is right? Should you vaccinate, and if so, when? And there are smaller ones: Is swaddling actually a good idea? Does your baby need a schedule right away?

These questions don't die out as your child ages, either. Sleeping and eating just start to stabilize, and then you'll get your first tantrum. What on earth do you do with that? Should you discipline your kid? How? Exorcism? Sometimes it seems like it. You may just need a break for a minute. Is it okay to let the kid watch TV? Maybe one time the internet told you watching TV will turn your child into a serial killer. It's difficult to remember the details—but maybe don't risk it? But, boy, a break would be nice.

And on top of these questions is the endless worrying, "Is my kid normal?" When your baby is just a few weeks old, "normal" is whether they are peeing enough, crying too much, gaining enough weight. Then it's how much they sleep, whether they roll over, whether they smile. Then do they crawl, do they walk, when do they run? And can they talk? Do they say enough different words?

How can we get the answers to these questions? How do we know the "right" way to parent? Does such a thing even exist? Your pediatrician will be helpful, but they tend to (correctly) focus on areas of actual medical concern. When my daughter showed no interest in walking at fifteen months, the doctor simply told me that if she didn't walk by eighteen months, we would start screening for developmental delay. But whether your child is so delayed that they need early intervention is different from whether they are simply a bit slower than the average. And it doesn't tell you if late milestones have any consequences.

At a more basic level, your doctor isn't always around. It's three a.m.

and your three-week-old will only sleep while you're right next to him. Is it okay to have him sleep in your bed? In this day and age, you're most likely to turn to the internet. Bleary-eyed, holding the baby, your partner (what an asshole—this is all their fault anyway) snoring next to you, you look through websites, parenting advice, Facebook feeds.

This can leave you worse off than you were before. There's no lack of opinions on the internet, and many of them are from people you probably trust—your friends, mommy bloggers, people who claim to know the research. But they all say different things. Some of them tell you that, yes, having your baby sleep in your bed is great. It's the natural way to do it, and there's no risk as long as you don't smoke or drink. They make a case that the people who say it's risky are just confused; they're thinking about people who don't do this the "right way."

But, on the other hand, the official recommendations say to *definitely not do this*. Your child could die. There is no safe way to co-sleep. The American Academy of Pediatrics tells you to put the baby in the bassinet next to your bed. He wakes up immediately.

This is all made worse by the fact that these comments are (often) not delivered in a calm manner. I have witnessed many an intense Facebook group discussion in which a decision about sleep deteriorates into, effectively, judgment about who is a good parent. You'll have people telling you that choosing to co-sleep isn't just a bad decision, it's one that would be made by someone who *doesn't care about their baby at all*.

In the face of all this conflicting information, how can you decide what is right not just for the baby, not just for you, but for your family overall? This is the crucial question of parenting.

I'm an economist; a professor whose work focuses on health economics. In my day job I analyze data, trying to tease causality out of the relationships I study. And then I try to use that data inside some economic framework—one that thinks carefully about costs and benefits—to think about decision-making. I do this in my research, and it's the focus of my teaching.

I also try to use these principles in decision-making outside the office and classroom. It probably helps that my husband, Jesse, is also an econo-mist: since we speak the same language, it gives us a framework to make family decisions together. We tend to use economics a lot in the household, and new parenting was no exception.

For example: Before we had Penelope, I used to cook dinner most nights. It was something I really enjoyed doing, and a relaxing way to end the day. We'd eat late—seven thirty or eight—then relax a bit and go to sleep.

When Penelope first arrived, we stuck to this schedule. But once she was old enough to eat with us, things got crazy. She needed to eat at six, and we arrived home (at best) at five forty-five. We wanted to eat together, but what kind of food can you prep and cook in fifteen minutes?

Cooking from scratch at the end of the day was an impossible chal-lenge. I considered the other options. We could get take-out. We could make two meals—a quick one for Penelope and a more involved one for us once she was in bed. Around this time I also learned about the concept of the meal kit: Pre-prepped ingredients for a set recipe—all you have to do is cook. There was even a vegetarian version that would deliver to our house.

With all these options, how do you choose?

If you want to think about this like an economist, you've got to start with data. In this case, the important question was: How does the cost of these choices compare to meal planning and prepping on my own? Get-ting take-out was more expensive. Feeding Penelope chicken nuggets and eating on our own was similar. The meal kits were somewhere in the middle: slightly more expensive than buying the same ingredients and preparing them myself, but less expensive than take-out.

But this wasn't the whole story, since this didn't take into account the value of my time. Or, as economists like to say, the "opportunity cost." I was spending time prepping food—fifteen, thirty minutes a day, usually early in the morning. I could have spent it doing something else (say, writ-ing my first book more quickly, or writing more papers). This time had real value, and we couldn't ignore it in the calculation.

Once we factored this in, the meal kit seemed like a great deal, and even take-out started to sound appealing. The dollar difference was small, and the cost of my time more than made up for it. Cooking two dinners, though, looked a lot worse: more time cooking, not less.

And yet this is still not quite right, since it doesn't account for preferences. I might really like to meal plan and prep—many people do. In this case, it might make sense to cook, even if another option seems like a good deal on the cost side. Basically, I might be willing (in economic terms) to "pay" something for the choice to cook.

Although take-out may be the easiest option in terms of time, some families really value a home-cooked meal. And in thinking about the two-dinner option, some parents want to sit and eat together with their kids every night, and others like the idea of a child dinner and a separate adult dinner, a chance to relax and chat with your spouse. Or maybe you like a mix of these.

Preferences are very important here. Two families—with the same food costs, the same value of time, the same options—may make different choices because they have different preferences. This economic approach to decision-making doesn't make a choice for you, only tells you how to structure it.

It tells you to ask questions like, how much would you need to enjoy cooking to make that the right choice?

For us, we wanted to eat with Penelope, and we didn't like the take-out options available. I decided that although I do like to cook, I didn't like it enough to want to do the whole process myself, so we tried the vegetarian meal kit (it was good—slightly heavy on the kale).

This household example may seem divorced from a choice like whether to breastfeed, but in terms of how to make the decision, it's not so different. You need the data—in this case, good information about the benefits of breastfeeding—and you also need to think about your family preferences.

When I was pregnant with Penelope, I brought this approach to bear on pregnancy. I wrote a book—*Expecting Better*—analyzing the many rules of pregnancy and the statistics behind them.

When Penelope was born, the decisions didn't stop—they just got harder. There was now an actual person to contend with, and even as a baby, she had opinions. You want your kid to be happy all the time! And yet you have to balance this with knowing that sometimes you need to make hard choices for them.

Consider, for example, Penelope's affinity for the Rock 'n Play Sleeper, which is a rocking bassinet-seat contraption. In the wake of the swaddle, Penelope decided that this was her sleep location of choice. This was at best inconvenient—we dragged that sleeper everywhere for months, including on a somewhat ill-planned vacation to Spain—and at worst generated a risk for a flattened head.

And yet extricating ourselves from that required not just us, but her. When we decided one day that we were done with it, she didn't nap for an entire day, leaving her a cranky mess and our nanny distraught. Penelope won that round; we returned to the sleeper the next day, only to finally be forced to give it up when she was above the weight limit.

Now, you could say we just gave in, but really, we made a decision to prioritize family harmony over moving Penelope to her crib exactly at the moment the books recommended. There are lines you shouldn't cross with young children, but there are many more gray areas. Thinking about our choices in cost/benefit terms helps take some of the stress off a decision.

In thinking about these decisions, I again, as I had during pregnancy, found there was comfort in starting with the data. For most of the larger decisions we had to make—breastfeeding, sleep training, allergies—there were studies. Of course, the trouble was that not all of these studies were very good.

Take breastfeeding. Breastfeeding is often hard, but you'll hear endlessly about the benefits. Breastfeeding is made out to be an absolute must by the medical establishment and a host of online voices, to say nothing of your friends and family. But are these benefits all real?

It's actually not so easy to answer that question.

The goal of studying breastfeeding is to see if children who are breastfed are different later in life—healthier, smarter—than those who are not.

The basic problem is that most people do not choose to breastfeed at random. In fact, people think carefully about this choice, and the kind of people who choose to do it are different from those who do not. When we look at recent data from the US, breastfeeding is more common among women with more education and higher income.

This is partly because these women are more likely to have the support (including maternity leave) that affords them the ability to breastfeed. It also may be partly because they're more aware of the recommendations that say that the choice to breastfeed is a crucial part of raising a healthy and successful child. But regardless of the reason, the fact remains.

This is a problem for learning from the data. Studies of breastfeeding show time and again that breastfeeding is associated with better outcomes for kids—better school performance, lower obesity rates, and so on. But these outcomes are also linked with a mother's education, income, and marital status. How can we know if it is the breastfeeding or the other differences among women that causes the better school performance and lower obesity?

One answer is that some of the data is better than other data.

In thinking about these decisions, I used my economic training—especially the part where I try to tease causality out of data—to try to separate the good studies from the less-good ones. Causality isn't simple. It can look like there is a strong relationship between two things, but when you dig a bit deeper, you find they aren't related at all. For instance, people who eat Clif Bars are likely healthier than those who don't. This probably isn't because of the Clif Bars, but rather that the people who choose to eat them are engaging in other healthy behaviors.

A large part of my approach here was to try to identify which of the hundreds of breastfeeding studies provided the best data.

Sometimes when I did this, the best studies did support a relationship—breastfeeding does, for example, seem to consistently reduce infant diarrhea. But at other times, the best studies didn't show these effects; the idea that breastfeeding has dramatic effects on IQ, for example, isn't as convincing.

In the case of breastfeeding, there are studies to rely on, even if they aren't all great. But even this isn't always true. When my kids were a bit older and I wondered about the effects of screen time, I found precious little data that really addressed the questions I had. IPad apps to teach a three-year-old letters simply haven't been around long enough to have prompted lots of research papers.

This was occasionally frustrating, but it is comforting, in its own way, to know there are some questions data just cannot answer for you. At least you can go into this with an understanding of the uncertainties.

As with the meal preparation question, data is only one piece of the puzzle, and we can't stop there. When I saw the data, I made one set of choices. But the same data does not always lead everyone to the same decision. Data is an input, but so are preferences. In deciding whether to breastfeed, it is useful to know what the benefits are (if any), but it's also crucial to think about the costs. You may hate breastfeeding; you may plan to return to work and hate pumping. These are reasons not to breast-feed. Too often we focus on the benefits at the expense of thinking about the costs. But benefits can be overstated, and costs can be profound.

These preferences, it should be noted, should consider not just the baby but also the parents. In thinking about the right caregiving setup for your child—stay-at-home parent, day care, nanny—it's useful to look at the data, but it is also crucial to think about what works for your family. In my case, I was committed to getting back to work. Perhaps my children would have preferred I stay home (I doubt it), but that wasn't going to work for *me*. I did get some data to think about this decision, but ultimately, my preferences played an important role. I made an informed choice, but I also made the choice that was right for me.

This idea—that what parents need or want will play a role in choices—can be hard to admit. In a sense, I think this is at the core of a lot of the "Mommy War" conflicts.

We all want to be good parents. We want our choices to be the right ones. So, after we make the choices, there is a temptation to decide they *are* the perfect ones. Psychology has a name for this: avoiding cognitive dissonance. If I choose not to breastfeed, I don't want to acknowledge that there are even small possible benefits to breastfeeding. So I encamp myself in the position that breastfeeding is a waste of time. On the other side, if I spend two years taking my boobs out every three hours, I need to believe that this is what it takes to deliver a life of continued successes to my child.

This is a deeply human temptation, but it is also really counterproductive. Your choices can be right for you but also not necessarily the best choices for other people. Why? *You are not other people.* Your circumstances differ. Your preferences differ. In the language of economics, your constraints differ.

When economists talk about people making the "optimal choices," we're always solving problems of what we call "constrained optimization." Sally likes apples and bananas. Apples cost $3 and bananas cost $5. Before we ask how many of each Sally buys, we give her a budget. This is her constraint. Otherwise, she'd buy infinite apples and bananas (economists assume people always want more stuff).

When we make parenting choices, we are also constrained—in money, yes, but also in time or energy. You can't make up sleep out of thin air. If you sleep less, you're giving up the benefits you may derive from a good night's sleep. That time spent pumping in the lactation room at work could be spent working. You think about this, and then you make the choices that work for you. But someone who needs less sleep, or has more time to nap, or can pump and work at the same time—they may make different choices. Parenting is hard enough. Let's take some of the stress out of parenting decisions.

This book will not tell you what decisions to make for your kids. Instead, I'll try to give you the necessary inputs and a bit of a decision framework. The data is the same for us all, but the decisions are yours alone.

In thinking through the big choices of these early years, you'll probably find that some of the data, on everything from sleep to screen time, is a surprise here. There is reassurance in seeing the numbers for yourself.

People may tell you it's fine to let your child "cry it out" to fall asleep, but you'll probably feel better doing it once you've seen the data shows this to be true.

When I wrote *Expecting Better*, about pregnancy, there was a lot of data—on coffee, alcohol, prenatal testing, epidurals. Preferences played an important role there, but in many cases, the data was clear. For example: Bed rest is not a good idea. Relative to pregnancy, there are fewer things here where the data will tell you what to do or avoid. Your family preferences will be more central. This doesn't mean the data isn't helpful—it often is!—but the decisions that come out of data will be different, even more so than they are in pregnancy.

Cribsheet starts in the delivery room. The first part of the book will cover some of the issues—many of them medical—that will come up early on: circumcision, newborn screening tests, infant weight loss. I'll talk about the early weeks at home: Should you swaddle? Avoid germ exposure? Obsessively collect data about your baby? This part of the book will also talk about the physical recovery from childbirth for birth moms, and about awareness of postpartum emotional issues.

Part 2 is focused on the big decisions of early parenting: breastfeeding (Should you do it? How does it work?), vaccinations, sleep position, sleep training, staying at home versus working outside the home, day care versus nanny. (Basically, the Mommy Wars.)

Part 3 will tackle the transition from baby to toddler, or at least a piece of it: screen time (good or bad?), potty training, discipline, and various educational choices. I'll show you some data on when your kid will walk and run, and how much they will talk (and whether it matters).

Finally, the last part of the book talks parents. When a baby arrives, it necessarily creates parents, and a lot will change. I'll talk about the stresses early parenting can have on your relationship with your partner, and the question of having more children (and when).

We know being a parent means getting a lot of advice, but this advice is almost never accompanied by an explanation of *why* something is true or not, or to what degree we can even know it's true. And by not explaining why, we remove people's ability to think about these choices for them-selves, with their own preferences playing a role. Parents are people, too, and they deserve better.

The goal of this book is not to fight against any particular piece of ad-vice but against the idea of not explaining why. Armed with the evidence and a way to think about decisions, you can make choices that are right for *your* family. If you're happy with your choices, that's the path to happier and more relaxed parenting. And, hopefully, to a bit more sleep.

PART ONE

In the Beginning

Regardless of whether you had the childbirth you always imagined or, in the words of a colleague, "got a little panicked at the end," you will find yourself in a recovery room a few hours later. It'll probably be pretty similar to your labor and delivery room, only when you arrived in *that* room, there was one fewer person along for the ride.

It is hard to overstate how different things are in the moments before and after the baby, especially when that baby is your first child. After Penelope was born, we were in the hospital for a few days. I sat around in a bathrobe, trying to nurse, holding the baby, waiting for her to be brought back from various tests, trying gently to walk around. Some memories of that time are very sharp and specific—Jane and Dave came with a purple stuffed bear, Aude brought a baguette—but the experience seems a bit like a dream.

In Jesse's notes about the first few days of Penelope's life, he wrote, "Emily wants to stare at the baby all the time." It's true. Even when I tried to sleep, I could see her behind my eyes.

The first few hours or days in the hospital, and then the first weeks at home, can have a kind of hazy quality. (This might be the sleep deprivation.) You're not seeing many other people (unless you're hosting unwelcome family members) or leaving the house much, you're not sleeping or eating enough, and there is all of a sudden a demanding person who wasn't there before. A WHOLE PERSON. Someone who will one day drive a car and have a job and tell you they hate you for ruining their life for not letting them go to a coed sleepover that *everyone else* is going to.

But while you're staring at the baby or contemplating the meaning of life, some stuff might come up that you have to make decisions about. Better to think about it in advance, since this will not be your most functional period. The days right after giving birth are a confusing time, and can be made more so because of the often conflicting advice you will receive from your care providers, your family and friends, and the online world.

The first chapter in this section discusses issues that may come up at the hospital—either procedures you could have there or complications that could arise early on. The second chapter talks about the first weeks at home.

There are a lot of big decisions about parenting—breastfeeding, vaccination, sleep location—which you'll also probably want to make early on (or, in some cases, before birth). But since these affect much more than just these first weeks, I'll leave them for part 2.

The First Three Days

I f you have a vaginal delivery, you'll probably spend two nights in the hospital. If you have a caesarean section, or any complications during birth, this might be three or four nights. There was a time when women would stay in the hospital for a week or even ten days to recover after giving birth, but that time has decidedly ended. Insurance can be so strict about this that one friend suggested we try to wait to have the baby until after midnight to get another hospital overnight. (This presumed a level of control that I definitely didn't have, although sometimes doctors will check you in late for this reason.)

Depending on your temperament (and the hospital), this can be a nice way to start out, or it can be a little frustrating. The big advantage of the hospital is that there are people around to take care of you and to help you figure out things with the baby. There are usually lactation consultants, if you want to breastfeed, and there are nurses around to make sure you aren't bleeding too much and that the baby looks like it is functioning normally.

The disadvantage is that the hospital is not your home. You don't have any of your stuff, it can be a little stifling, and the food is typically terrible.

With Penelope, we spent the requisite two days at a big hospital in Chicago. We have one truly appalling photo of me from this period in which Jesse thought it would be funny to hold up a copy of *Us Weekly*, which had an article about Britney Spears entitled "My New Life," next to me and take a picture. Let's just say I was starting "my new life" with a really puffy face.

Most of this time, you'll just be sitting around, staring at your baby, posting status updates to Facebook. But occasionally someone will come in and want to do things to the baby. They'll roll in a giant machine for a hearing test. They'll do a heel prick to test the baby's blood. And sometimes they'll ask you what you want to do.

"Do you want us to circumcise him while you're here?"

How do you make a decision like this? It isn't an obvious one for many people. It's not a medically or legally required procedure. It's really up to you.

There are many ways to make choices in this situation. You can do what your friends do, or what your doctor recommends. You can try to figure out what people on the internet say they did, and why. Of course, in a situation like circumcision, this probably won't help you. About half of male babies in the US are circumcised, and about half are not, which means you can find plenty of people on either side of the issue. (Why is it half? Hard to know. Some people do this for religious reasons, others for medical reasons, some because the dad is circumcised and parents want their son's penis to look the same as Dad's.)

This book is going to argue for a more structured approach to making this choice. First, you get the data. You really confront—in an open-minded way—the question of whether there are any risks, and what these risks are. Are there any benefits? What and how big are they? Sometimes there are benefits to a choice, but they are so vanishingly small that it may not make sense to think about them very much. Likewise, sometimes there are risks, but they are infinitesimal relative to the other risks you take every day.

And then, second, you combine this evidence with your preferences. Is your extended family strongly in favor or not? Is it important to you that your son have a penis that looks like his dad's? There is no data to tell you the answers to these questions, but they're an important piece of the puzzle.

These preferences are why you really can't rely on that lady on the internet. She doesn't live with your family, and honestly, she has no idea what the right thing is for your kid's penis.

For the decisions you *can* plan, it's helpful to have thought them through in advance. The early period in the hospital is overwhelming, and not a great time for decision-making (although just wait until you get home!). It's good to be prepared so you know what's going on while you adapt to your "new life."

Usually, things go smoothly, and a couple of days after delivery, you'll be packing your baby into their car seat and heading out. But this is also a time when some common newborn complications creep in—jaundice, excess weight loss—and you may have to deal with them. These complications are good to be aware of in advance, which can help you be a more active participant in decisions related to them.

THE EXPECTED . . .

Newborn Baths

When the baby comes out, it is all covered in stuff. Not to get too graphic, but a lot of that is blood. There is some amniotic fluid, and a waxy covering called the vernix that protects the baby from infection in the womb. At some point, someone may suggest you wash the baby off.

I recall the nurse attempting to show us how to wash Penelope in an infant tub, probably a day or so after her birth. We watched carefully and then agreed among ourselves that it was impossible to do that and we'd probably just wait until she could do it herself. We made it two weeks, at which point we finally gave in to the spoiled milk in her balled-up fists. We memorialized this bath in pictures of a totally panicked infant who probably has still not forgiven us.

But I digress.

It used to be common to wash the baby immediately—like, within the first few minutes, perhaps even before it was handed off to Mom. There is now some pushback against this for two reasons. First, there is an increasing trend toward immediate skin-to-skin contact (more on that below) and toward leaving Mom and baby alone for a couple of hours right after birth. One of the benefits of skin-to-skin contact seems to be increased breastfeeding success. Perhaps for this reason, breastfeeding success also seems to be increased by delaying the bath past the first few hours.[1] Since there is no actual reason to give the baby a bath, this is a perfectly sensible reason to delay.

The other concern about early bathing is that it may affect infant temperature. When they are first born, infants sometimes have trouble maintaining their body temperature. Bathing them—and then, more important, taking them out of the bath wet—is hypothesized to have some negative impacts on this process. This turns out not to be well supported in the data. In studies that look at bathing *immediately* after birth, there are no sustained consequences for the baby's temperature.[2]

There does seem to be some evidence that infants given sponge baths in particular experience more temperature variability in the short term— i.e., during the bath and very immediately after.[3] There's just more time when the wet, naked infant is exposed to the air. Temperature variability is not so much a problem in itself, but it could be misinterpreted as a sign of infection. This could lead to other unnecessary interventions. For this reason, tub baths are the mode of choice in most hospitals.

So a bath isn't a terrible thing, but there is also really no reason to bathe your kid other than some gross-out factor. Most of the blood can just kind of be wiped off. I should perhaps not admit this, but they never bathed Finn in the hospital at all, and we still waited the family-standard two weeks to actually give him a bath at home. Nothing bad happened as a result, and given Finn's reaction when we did it, Jesse still feels we should have waited longer.

Circumcision

Male circumcision is a procedure in which the foreskin of the penis is removed surgically. Circumcision is documented as long ago as ancient Egypt, and is practiced widely by many different societies. It's not clear why this arose; there are a variety of theories—my favorite of which is that some leader was born without a foreskin and therefore made everyone else remove theirs—and the practice might have begun for different reasons in different locations.

Circumcision can be performed at various ages, and in some cultures is traditionally done at puberty as part of an initiation ritual. In the US, however, if a boy is circumcised, it is typically shortly after birth. For people who practice Judaism, circumcisions are done in a ritual called a bris when the baby is eight days old. Outside a traditional bris, your child may be circumcised before they leave the hospital, or as an outpatient procedure a few days later. In principle, circumcision can be done more or less as soon as you can confirm that the penis is working properly (i.e., after the first time the kid pees).

Circumcision is an optional procedure. It's not common everywhere—for example, Europeans typically do not circumcise. It has historically been quite common in the US, although circumcision rates have declined some over time, from an estimated 65 percent of births in 1979 to 58 percent in 2010.

If you are part of a religious group in which this is traditionally done, you'll very likely circumcise your child. For people outside this set, there is a healthy debate about whether circumcision is a good idea. There are those who strongly oppose it, feeling it is a risky form of mutilation, and those who support it, arguing in favor of health benefits. The conversation can get heated, so it helps to see the data.

The major risk from circumcision, like any surgical procedure, is infection. For infant circumcisions performed in a hospital, these risks are very small. The most comprehensive estimates suggest that perhaps 1.5 percent of infant circumcisions result in minor complications, and virtually none result in serious adverse complications.[4] These figures are based on studies that include some developing countries, so even the minor adverse consequences are likely to be less frequent in the US.

Another risk is what is sometimes called "poor aesthetic outcome"— basically, residual foreskin that will require further surgery. There aren't great estimates of how common this is, although it seems to be somewhat more common than the overall rate of adverse complications.[5]

Very rarely, babies can develop meatal stenosis, a condition in which the urethra (the tube through which urine passes) is compressed, making it hard to pee. This is more common in circumcised than uncircumcised boys, making it fairly clear that the condition is associated with circumcision, but again, the condition is extremely rare overall.[6] Repairing meatal stenosis is possible, but requires a second surgery. There is some limited evidence that it may be prevented by slathering Vaseline (or Aquaphor) on the penis for the baby's first six months.[7]

There is also some discussion—especially in the anticircumcision camp—about loss of penis sensitivity as a result of circumcision. There simply isn't any evidence for this either way. Small studies of penile sensitivity (conducted by poking the penis with stuff) do not show any consistent results on circumcised versus uncircumcised men.[8] The researchers also likely deduced that no one likes to have their penis poked, intact foreskin or not.

This covers the risks. There are also some possible benefits to circumcision. The first is the prevention of urinary tract infections (UTIs). Circumcised boys are much less likely to get these. About 1 percent of uncircumcised boys will get a UTI during childhood. For circumcised boys, the estimate is just 0.13 percent.[9] This is highly significant, and it is generally accepted that this protection is real. However, it is worth saying that the benefit is small in absolute terms: you'd have to circumcise one hundred boys to prevent one UTI.

Uncircumcised boys can also develop a condition called phimosis, where it becomes impossible to pull the foreskin back. This will need treatment—typically with a steroid cream—and possibly require a circumcision at an older age. The overall risk of needing a later circumcision for this condition (or related ones) is estimated at 1 to 2 percent—so, rare, but not unheard of.[10]

The last two cited benefits of circumcision are a lower risk of HIV and other sexually transmitted infections (STIs) and a lower risk of penile cancer. In the case of HIV and other STIs, there is good evidence from a number of countries in Africa suggesting risks are lower for circumcised men. This is in a context where most transmission of HIV is heterosexual; in the US, most transmission is through men who have sex with men (this is the technical jargon) or through IV drug use. It is unclear from the data whether the circumcision protections extend to cases of men having sex with men—they certainly do not to IV drug use.[11]

Penile cancer is extremely rare—affecting an estimated 1 in 100,000 men. The risk of invasive penile cancer increases with lack of circumcision, especially among boys who had phimosis as a child.[12] Again, however, even a large increase in the relative risk translates to a tiny number of cases.

The American Academy of Pediatrics suggests the health benefits of circumcision outweigh the costs, but they note correctly that both benefits and costs are quite small. This decision will often come down to personal preference, some type of cultural linkage, or just a desire to have your son's penis look a particular way. These are all valid reasons to do it or not do it.

If you do choose to circumcise, there is the consideration of pain relief. People used to believe that small babies didn't experience pain the way adults do, and as a result it was common to do circumcisions with no pain relief treatment—or maybe just some sugar water. This is wrong, and indeed, it seems that infants who experience pain during circumcision have a worse reaction to pain from vaccinations even four to six months later.[13]

In light of this, it is now strongly recommended that infants have some type of pain relief during this procedure. The most effective type seems to be a penile nerve block (typically called a DPNB), which involves injecting a painkiller into the base of the penis before the circumcision. Your baby's doctor may also use topical anesthetic in combination.[14]

Blood and Hearing Tests

The medical staff at the hospital will take advantage of the time you're there to do at least two additional tests on your baby: a blood screening and a hearing test.

The newborn blood screening is used to test for a very wide variety of conditions. Depending on the state, the exact number varies; California (for example) is on the high end, with sixty-one. Many of these conditions relate to metabolism and test for inability to digest particular proteins or produce enzymes.

A good example—likely the most common disorder detected in this way—is phenylketonuria (PKU). PKU is a genetic condition that affects about 1 in 10,000 births. People with this condition lack a particular enzyme that breaks down the amino acid phenylalanine into another amino acid. For people with PKU, eating a low-protein diet is crucial, since protein contains a lot of phenylalanine. In a person with PKU, protein can build up in the body, including in the brain, and cause extremely serious complications, including severe intellectual disability and death.

Once PKU is detected, however, dietary modifications make it extremely manageable and the negative consequences can be avoided. The problem is that if PKU is not detected at birth, brain damage can occur pretty much immediately, since breast milk and formula both have significant amounts of protein. Without testing, you wouldn't know until too late.

Testing for this condition—and others like it—at birth is therefore crucial to improve prognosis. These tests are all done with a small heel prick, and there is no risk to the baby. If your child doesn't have any of these conditions (by far the most likely scenario), you will not hear anything more about it.

Medical staff will also do a hearing test on the baby, which involves a large and complicated machine; sometimes this is wheeled into your room and the test is conducted there, other times in another location. Hearing loss is relatively common, affecting perhaps 1 to 3 in 1,000 children. There is an increasing emphasis on early detection of hearing loss, as early intervention (for example, with hearing aids or implants) can improve language acquisition and decrease the need for intervention later.

As you might imagine, you cannot run a hearing test on an infant as you would on an adult—babies don't raise their hands when they hear a beep, and honestly, they're probably asleep anyway. Instead, these tests use sensors on the head or ear probes. The sensors or probes can detect whether the middle and inner ear are responding as expected to a tone.[15]

These tests are quite good at detecting hearing loss (they catch 85 to 100 percent of cases), but turn up a lot of false positives. By some estimates, 4 percent of infants will fail this test, while only 0.1 to 0.3 percent actually have hearing loss. A failed hearing test will typically generate a referral to a formal audiological center, which is a good idea given the need to catch hearing problems early. But it's also a good idea to remember that most babies who fail this do not have hearing problems; if your baby fails on the first round, it may be a good idea to try again while you're in the hospital, as a second test can catch some false positives.

Rooming In

During these first days in the hospital, you'll see a lot of your baby. There is a question, however, of whether you want to be with them every minute. Childbirth is exhausting, and for many women, sleeping with their infant in their room is hard. Hospital nurseries have, historically, provided a way for women to take a break from their babies to recover and rest for a few hours.

However, this is no longer as true as it once was. In the past few decades, we've seen the rise of "baby-friendly hospitals." Obviously, one would hope that all hospitals are baby friendly, but the baby-friendly hospital designation means something more specific. In particular, baby-friendly hospitals must follow a ten-point plan designed to improve breastfeeding.

These tenets include things like not giving infants formula unless medically indicated, not giving pacifiers, and informing all pregnant women about the benefits of breastfeeding. I won't go into the breastfeeding part here, as there's much more on that later in the book. And the practice of avoiding pacifiers, which is especially controversial, will also get more treatment in the chapter on breastfeeding.

But in addition to advice and avoidance of formula, one of the requirements of baby-friendly hospitals is that they must practice "rooming in." That is, unless there is a medical reason the infant has to be out of the room, mothers and babies should be together in their room twenty-four hours a day.

This might seem great to you! Why would you want to be away from your baby? And, indeed, it can be lovely. When I had Finn, I ended up in a birthing room with a giant bed, and they let us stay there for an entire day (thanks, Women and Infants Hospital!). There was enough space for both Jesse and me to be in the bed, taking turns sleeping, with Finn between us. I think back on this as a really amazing twelve-hour start to Finn's life.

On the other hand, this was somewhat unusual. More likely, you're in a recovery room with the baby in a bassinet next to you, a much less comfortable setup. Babies make a lot of weird noises, and having them with you all the time—well, you may not be able to sleep at all. Before I had Penelope, more than one fellow mom told me to just send her to the nursery—even for a few hours—so I could get some sleep. (Which I did— Prentice Hospital in Chicago did not qualify as baby friendly at the time.)

There is some disagreement about the wisdom of rooming-in recommendations as policy. It's always tricky to think about policies that rely on rules that effectively remove patients' choices. On the other hand, there's some evidence that this is very beneficial for some women—for example, those whose babies have neonatal abstinence syndrome (a result of maternal use of opioids during pregnancy)—so there are reasons to encourage both women and hospitals to do it.

From the standpoint of this book, however, I'm not interested in commenting on policy, but rather on what the data says you should do if you are given a choice. This choice could be in the form of rooming in or not, if you're in a hospital that isn't baby friendly, or it could be the choice of hospital in the first place.

There is a clear trade-off: rooming in will mean less sleep, but maybe it's good for the baby. This is your first sleep test. Is rooming in beneficial enough to warrant some lost sleep in the first days? To answer this, we need to know more about the size of the benefits. And for that, we need the data.

The main purported benefit of rooming in is improved breastfeeding success. There really isn't much evidence supporting this benefit. There are clearly correlations: women who keep their infant with them are more likely to breastfeed, but this is hard to interpret as causal since these women differ in other ways. Most notably, women who *want* to breastfeed may be more likely to keep their infant with them to try to figure out how to do it. The breastfeeding might cause the rooming in, rather than the rooming in causing the breastfeeding.

To the extent that we have any evidence, the results are mixed. On one hand, in a large study conducted in Switzerland comparing the breastfeeding outcomes for babies born in baby-friendly hospitals there versus those born elsewhere, the authors found more breastfeeding for babies born in these hospitals. On the other hand, it's hard to know if this is the result of rooming in or something else.[16] These hospitals were different in many ways, and the study has no way to control for who *chooses* this type of hospital, which is likely linked to breastfeeding intentions.

In studying questions like this, the "gold standard" way to draw conclusions is with a randomized trial. Here's how that would work in this case: First, we'd take a group of women and randomly pick half of them to do rooming in; the other half would not, but otherwise, we'd treat them the same. Since we picked the groups randomly, we can be confident in drawing conclusions by comparing them. If the rooming-in group has higher breastfeeding rates, then we should attribute that to the rooming in. On the other hand, if the breastfeeding rates are not different, this suggests there may not be a relationship.

In the case of rooming in, there is one randomized trial of 176 women studying this question. It is not very encouraging. The study finds no impact on breastfeeding at six months, and no impact on the median time of breastfeeding.[17] This study does find some increase in breastfeeding at four days of life, although it is a bit hard to interpret since the researchers encouraged feeding on a fixed schedule for some groups and not others.

It would be hard to argue that the data strongly supports the breastfeeding benefits of rooming in; at best we can say that we can't rule out *some* effects. But you'll hear from hospitals who advocate rooming in that there's no reason *not* to do this, so we should do it even if the benefits are uncertain.

This is not, however, entirely true: there may be a very good reason *not* to choose rooming in. In the days after giving birth, women are often very tired. Your hospital stay includes more support than you are likely to get at home, and sending your baby to the nursery could let you take advantage of their expert care of you and your baby. Knowing that the data is not definitively on the side of rooming in can make this an easier choice for some moms.

Additionally, there could actually be some (small) risks to rooming in. Many women fall asleep while breastfeeding; this is more likely the more tired you are, and not getting a break to sleep can contribute to the risk that an infant could be seriously hurt as a result of an exhausted mom falling asleep with the baby.[18] There are also safety concerns about bed sharing in general, whether in the hospital or at home (more on this in the chapter on sleep location).

A 2014 paper on this issue reported on eighteen cases of infant death or near death as a result of hospital bed sharing.[19] This research is not equipped to comment on overall risk levels; their goal was simply to collect case reports of this to show it was a possibility.

Another study reported that 14 percent of babies born in baby-friendly hospitals were "at risk of" falling from the bed, mostly due to their mothers falling asleep while nursing.[20] Just to be clear, this wasn't 14 percent of infants falling, just those that nurses felt were *at risk of* falling.

In my view, the most important thing to come out of this is, if you have the option to send your kid to the nursery for a few hours and you want to do that, you shouldn't feel shame in doing so. There is no good evidence that you're disrupting your breastfeeding relationship, if that's important to you. And if you find yourself falling asleep with your baby in the bed, ask for help.

. . . AND THE UNEXPECTED

Infant Weight Loss

Many new parents are not expecting the tremendous focus doctors and hospital staff place on infant weight gain or loss. If you have (happily) given birth to a healthy baby after a relatively uneventful delivery, the vast majority of your hospital conversations will now revolve around the baby's feeding and weight. Obviously, you want your baby to thrive, and weight is an important metric of this. But when you're just postpartum and trying to breastfeed for the first time, this can be a very fraught conversation. It can feel like you are failing—you did such a great job growing this baby inside you, and now that it's out, you totally suck. (You don't! That's just how it feels.)

Infant weight is monitored pretty carefully in the hospital. Every twelve hours or so they'll weigh the baby and possibly come back to report any change in weight to you. On day 2 after I'd given birth to Penelope, they returned her to me at two a.m. and informed me she had lost 11 percent of her body weight and that we had to start supplementing right away. I was alone, bleary and confused, and ill-prepared to make a decision about this. The lessons from this are that you shouldn't let your husband go home to sleep, and, possibly secondary, that it's good to know this is a risk.

Given the focus on weight, it's important to be prepared. Here is the first thing to know: nearly all infants lose weight after birth, and those who are breastfed lose even more. The mechanisms for this are well understood. In the womb, your baby is getting nutrients and absorbing calories through the umbilical cord. Once the baby is out, he has to figure out how to eat. It is complicated (for both of you), and in the first few days, you won't yet have a lot of milk. Colostrum may or may not be the magical substance that lactation consultants fantasize about, but there isn't much of it (especially with your first baby).

The fact that this weight loss is expected means you want to be careful about this issue, but you also want to make sure not to overreact to the design of the system.

The reasons for weight monitoring are good ones. Weight loss is not an issue in and of itself, but excessive weight loss can indicate a problem with feeding—that breastfeeding isn't working successfully, for example. This can be a clue that newborns aren't getting enough liquid, which puts them at risk for dehydration. Dehydrated babies may then struggle more to feed, and you get a downward spiral. In principle this can have severe consequences, but these are rare.

Monitoring weight is about catching possible problems early, when you can fix them, and effective monitoring requires understanding how much weight newborns typically lose. Generally, we want to consider something a problem if it's way outside the normal range. There is nothing in biology that tells you that a baby losing, say, 10 percent of its birth weight is a trigger for problems. If most babies lose 10 percent of their weight, then we shouldn't worry when one does.

Figuring out the range of normal newborn weight loss requires data that, until recently, hasn't been that easy to come by. In 2015, however, a set of authors published a really nice paper in the journal *Pediatrics* that used data from hospital records on 160,000 births to graph out the weight loss among breastfed infants in the hours after birth.[21]

You can see a version of the study's graphs for the babies who were breastfed (more on formula feeding on page 20). The authors differentiate between infants born vaginally and those born by caesarean section. The horizontal axis shows infant age in hours; the vertical axis shows the percentage of weight loss. The lines indicate how much this varies. The top line, for example, shows the weight loss path over time for the baby at the 50th percentile of weight loss.

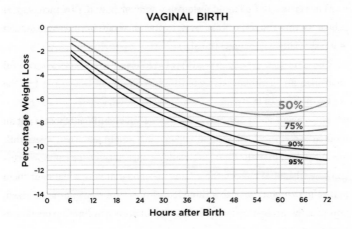

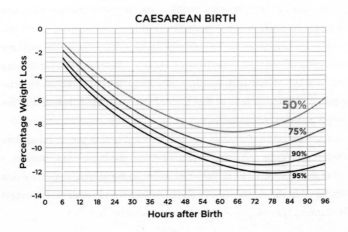

From these figures, you can read the average weight loss and the range. For example, at 48 hours, the average infant born vaginally has lost 7 percent of their body weight, and 5 percent of infants have lost more than 10 percent. For at least some infants, weight loss continues through 72 hours.

On average, babies born by caesarean section do seem to lose a bit more weight initially. Note that the C-section graph looks at a longer time frame than the vaginal birth graph, since these babies are typically in the hospital longer (due to Mom's recovery time).

What is this useful for? Mainly, this lets doctors (and, in principle, parents) evaluate where the child's weight loss is relative to the average, and thus ask if they are outside the norm. This graph tells us that if a baby is born by C-section, we can expect them to lose a bit more weight, so if they do, it shouldn't necessarily trigger an intervention.

The authors of this paper created a website, www.newbornweight.org, where you can enter the time of birth of your child, method of birth, method of feeding, birth weight, and current weight and learn where they are in the distribution.

When I had Penelope, the rule in the hospital was if the baby loses more than 10 percent of their body weight, you supplement. But you can see from the graphs that whether this is a reasonable cutoff depends tremendously on when the measurement is taken and the baby's particular circumstances. At 72 hours, 10 percent weight loss is inside the normal range. At 12 hours, it would be a serious outlier.

These graphs all refer to breastfed infants. Formula-fed infants lose much less weight (unlike breast milk, it doesn't take any time for formula to "come in"). By comparison, while the average breastfed infant has lost 7 percent of their weight at 48 hours, the average formula-fed infant has lost only 3 percent. Weight loss of more than 7 or 8 percent is very rare in this group. The same authors who made the breastfeeding graphs made ones for formula feeding, and their website lets you do your own calculations.

If you do find, as I did, that your infant has gone over the weight loss limits, what should you do? Typically, hospitals will recommend supplementation with formula or possibly donor milk. Water or sugar water was common in the past, but this isn't a good idea.

If this happens, you may worry that this will make it harder to breastfeed—I definitely did. There isn't much evidence on this—it's hard to really isolate the impact of a small amount of supplementation. But to the extent that we know anything, we know there's *no reason* to think a short period of supplementing with formula should impact breastfeeding success (if that is your goal) in the long run.[22] Supplementation would rarely be recommended before 48 or 72 hours, so it's useful to pay attention to your baby's weight before that. If she's losing weight quickly, trying to figure out why may make sense.

A final note: The major concern about weight loss is that it is a signal of dehydration. But this is also something you can monitor directly. If your baby is peeing with some frequency and does not have a dry tongue, there's a very good chance he's not dehydrated. Conversely, if you see these signs, supplementation may be a good idea, even if there isn't too much weight loss.

The extensive focus on weight and feeding is enough to really scare a lot of new parents (myself included). The data here is reassuring in both directions. Some pretty substantial weight loss is totally normal, even expected. So don't panic. And if you do have to supplement, don't panic then, either.

Jaundice

With a first child, most of us are prepared to be a bit surprised by the whole experience. After all, you've never done it before. Even I, a tremendously neurotic person, knew things would come up that I didn't expect. For example, we failed to buy any clothes that would leave the umbilical cord exposed while it healed. Emergency runs to Target were common.

With a second child, it's easier to feel like you know what you're doing. Before Finn, I felt prepared. I had the correct clothes. I had the bassinet. I was even ready with my weight loss data in case that came up (it didn't).

Surely I wouldn't unexpectedly face some medical or other issue with no preparation.

Obviously, this was ridiculous. Two days after we arrived home, I got a call from Finn's doctor: Finn had jaundice. I found myself rushing him back to the hospital in his infant bear snowsuit for another overnight stay. This mostly proves I do not learn from my overconfidence and will always be surprised by it.

Jaundice is a condition in which the liver is unable to fully process bilirubin, a by-product of breaking down red blood cells. Everyone, baby or not, relies on their liver to break these down, and in principle anyone can be jaundiced. Infants are at higher risk for this just after birth for a few reasons. There are more blood cells being broken down shortly after birth, increasing the load of bilirubin presented to the liver. At birth, the liver remains immature and therefore has difficulty excreting this higher load into the gut. Finally, in the first few days of life, babies are not eating a lot, so the bilirubin hangs out in the gut where it gets reabsorbed back into the bloodstream.

In high concentrations, bilirubin is neurotoxic (meaning it can poison the brain), so jaundice is potentially very serious in extreme cases. Severe untreated jaundice can lead to a condition called kernicterus, a form of long-term brain damage.

This is scary, and it's the reason jaundice is taken very seriously, but in virtually all cases, jaundice will not progress to kernicterus, even if untreated. Jaundice is also very common, especially in breastfed newborns: about 50 percent of newborns will have this condition to some degree. It's important to note that the brain injury effects are *not* on a continuum: at low or moderate concentrations, bilirubin doesn't cross the blood–brain barrier and is therefore not damaging.

To give a sense of the relative risks, there are two to four cases of kernicterus in the US each year. However, tens of thousands of children are treated for jaundice each week. Treatment protocols are extremely aggressive, and doctors are willing to treat many jaundiced babies who would be fine recovering on their own in order to avoid a single case of brain damage.

So while it is likely a good idea to undergo treatment if the guidelines suggest it, there is little reason to be worried about the worst-case scenario.

The primary sign of jaundice is that your baby's skin will turn yellow (this might also look more orange). The fact that your baby is yellow, however, doesn't necessarily mean they need treatment, and color on its own is not diagnostic. At Penelope's four-day visit, our pediatrician, Dr. Li, told us, "People will tell you she is yellow. Just ignore them."

In many babies, jaundice will simply resolve on its own as they eat and grow. Detecting whether jaundice has reached a problematic level requires testing. Many hospitals screen first with a special light that can estimate bilirubin levels through the skin, and use that to decide whether your baby needs a blood test to look at bilirubin levels in the blood. They may also skip straight to the blood test. This test doesn't need a lot of blood, so they'll typically use a heel prick to get a drop or two. The test results are reported in a number (11.4, say, or 16.1); higher numbers are worse.

Just as with weight loss, interpreting this test depends on the age of the baby. Bilirubin levels typically increase over the first few days after birth, so doctors will compare your baby's test results with the normal range for the number of hours old your child is.

The key decision for the doctor is whether bilirubin levels are high enough for "phototherapy"—aka a blue light box. This type of treatment typically occurs in the hospital, and involves having the infant spend time naked (other than a diaper and an eye covering) in a bassinet that is emitting blue fluorescent light. The light breaks down the bilirubin into other substances that are passed out of the body in the baby's urine.

Time in the box can be as little as a few hours or up to a few days (you take the baby out for feeding), depending on severity and how quickly the infant responds to the treatment. Daily (or more frequent) blood tests keep the doctor updated on how things are progressing.

In general, higher levels of bilirubin are worse—but how high is high enough to need treatment? The answer to this depends on the exact age of the baby in hours, and on their other features.

Specifically, doctors start by looking at whether your baby is low risk (more than 38 weeks of gestation, otherwise healthy), medium risk (36 to 38 weeks of gestation and healthy, or 38 or more weeks with other symptoms), or high risk (36 to 38 weeks of gestation with other symptoms). Once they have the risk level, doctors use graphs like the previous ones to decide whether the baby needs phototherapy. If the bilirubin levels are higher than the cutoffs, phototherapy is started. The following graph is for a low-risk baby. Here, for a baby 72 hours old, a number above 17 would suggest the need for treatment.[23] For higher-risk babies, the cutoffs are lower, and doctors intervene more aggressively.

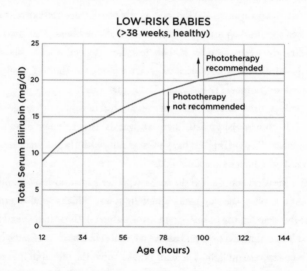

LOW-RISK BABIES
(>38 weeks, healthy)

As there is for determining risky infant weight loss, there is also a website that will tell you if jaundice treatment is recommended given bilirubin levels: www.bilitool.org. It's for doctors, but it's accessible to anyone who is curious.

It's worth noting that these guidelines do evolve over time, and as of this writing there is a push to make them more lenient and to treat jaundice less aggressively. If you find yourself in this situation, you may want to ask your doctor which guidelines they are using.

Very rarely, extremely severe or untreated cases of jaundice may need treatment beyond phototherapy. The final treatment option is an exchange transfusion, in which blood is simultaneously removed from the infant and replaced with a transfusion. This procedure can be lifesaving, although with good monitoring technology, it is very rarely necessary.

Jaundice is more common in some babies than others. Exclusively breastfed infants are more likely to develop it. Babies of Asian heritage are at higher risk. It is also more common when mothers and babies have different blood types. Rarely, there are underlying blood disorders that can exacerbate newborn jaundice.

Excessive newborn weight loss is a risk factor, as is bruising in delivery. In retrospect, our experience with Finn shouldn't have been as surprising as it was, since he got pretty banged up during delivery and came out all squashed and purple.

A NOTE: BACK IN THE DELIVERY ROOM

A few interventions occur right away when your baby arrives—typically before you even leave the delivery room. These include the possibility of delayed cord cutting, a vitamin K shot to promote better blood clotting, and an eye treatment to avoid possible complications from untreated sexually transmitted infections in the mother.

These interventions are covered in detail in the last chapter of *Expecting Better*. But since they do occur after birth, I'll review the conclusions here.

Delayed Cord Clamping

In the womb, the baby is attached to you with an umbilical cord. After birth, the cord is cut, but there is some debate over exactly when the cord should be cut: Do you cut right away, as is the standard practice? Or do you wait a few minutes for the baby to reabsorb some blood from the cord and then cut? This latter option is called "delayed cord cutting." The argument in favor of delaying is that the reabsorbed blood from the placenta is valuable.

For premature infants, there is very good evidence that you should delay cord clamping.[24] Randomized trials have shown improvements in blood volume, less anemia, and less need for transfusion as a result, among other outcomes.

For babies who are not premature, the evidence also largely favors delayed clamping, although it is slightly more mixed.[25] In particular, delaying cord clamping lowers the risk of anemia later and increases stores of iron, but also slightly increases the risk of jaundice.

On net, the recommendations increasingly favor delaying the cord cutting, if possible.

Vitamin K Shot

For decades, it has been standard practice to give a shot of vitamin K within the first hours after birth to prevent bleeding disorders. Too little vitamin K can cause unexpected bleeding in about 1.5 percent of infants in the first week of life, and is associated with rare but much more serious bleeding disorders later. Vitamin K supplementation can prevent bleeding.[26]

In the 1990s, there was a brief controversy about the possibility that this shot led to increased incidence of childhood cancer. The concern was based on very small studies, with suspect methods, and subsequent follow-up work rejected this link.[27] There are, therefore, no known risks to a vitamin K shot, but clear benefits from it. (Adam, my wonderful medical editor, begs you to please get the shot.)

Antibiotics in the Eye

If a mother has an untreated sexually transmitted infection—gonorrhea, in particular—and her child is born vaginally, there is a substantial risk of blindness as a result of infection. As a result, there is a policy of treating babies with antibiotic eye ointment as prophylaxis. This can prevent 85 to 90 percent of infections and does not have any recognized downsides.

The reasons for this treatment are increasingly less common, as all pregnant women are now tested and treated for STIs. And if you know you are not at risk, the antibiotics are unnecessary. You can opt out of this treatment in many states—easier in some than others—and this may be an option for you.

The Bottom Line

- Newborn baths early on are unnecessary, but not damaging. Tub baths are better than sponge baths.
- Circumcision has some small benefits and also carries some small risks. The choice is likely to come down largely to preference.
- Rooming in doesn't have any compelling effects on breastfeeding outcomes either way. It is worth being careful about falling asleep with your infant if you choose to keep them with you at all times.
- Infant weight loss should be monitored and compared with expectations; you can do this yourself at www.newborn weight.org.
- Jaundice is monitored with a blood test and should be treated if outside the normal range; you can monitor this yourself at www.bilitool.org.
- Delayed cord clamping is likely recommended, especially if your baby is premature. Vitamin K supplements are a good idea. Eye antibiotics are likely unnecessary for most babies but are mandated in some states and have no known downsides.

Wait, You Want Me to Take It Home?

I have two incredibly vivid memories from Penelope's first weeks at home. One is a moment around three weeks where I recall sitting on the couch in the basement, crying hysterically, after realizing I would never feel rested again. (This was only partially true.) But the first is of the moment we arrived. Penelope had fallen asleep on the way. We came through the back door. I was carrying the car seat. I put the seat down. And I remember thinking, *It's going to wake up. What do we do then?*

Perhaps because of this total uncertainty about what's going on (which, luckily, mostly lessens with later children), small concerns can totally take over. You are very tired, and you are now facing a challenge unlike any you have ever known. So cut yourself some slack if things get a little absurd.

For example, when we left the hospital, the doctors told us to keep mittens over Penelope's hands so she wouldn't scratch herself. But when my mother came to visit, she told us that if we did this, Penelope would never learn to use her hands.

In reflecting on this now, I cannot imagine why I was especially animated about this either way. But when I look back to my notes from that time, I find a paper entitled "Injury by Mittens in Neonates: A Report of an Unusual Presentation of This Easily Overlooked Problem and Literature Review."[1] Apparently this is the only paper I could find about mitten injuries, and it suggests a child can be injured by mittens, rather than that mittens prevent injury. The paper reports twenty cases of mitten injury since the 1960s, which, I think it's fair to say, makes this type of injury rare. I could not find anything that suggested mittens would prevent children from learning to use their hands.

I recall that we did stick with the mittens, despite the developmental concerns and injury risk. My mother had already lost some credibility earlier in her visit by insisting (in contrast to my doctor's advice) that I should limit how frequently I walked up and down the stairs.

It is beyond the scope of this book (or probably any book) to address all the crazy concerns that will come up in each particular case. And there are some questions I cannot answer—for example, is there any way to get infant poop stains out of white onesies? It's a question for the ages, and one we won't answer here.

In this chapter, I cover some concerns that come up right away: germ exposure, vitamin D drops, colic, and, finally, the value (or lack thereof) of data collection. These may seem mundane and minor. But they can loom very large for the brand-new parent.

Take for instance, the prisoner's dilemma, aka swaddling.

SWADDLING

When the nurses take your baby away at the hospital, it will invariably be returned tightly packed in a little blanket, swaddled up like a burrito. The hospital-grade swaddle is a baby straitjacket. No baby can escape it.

They'll probably send you home with a couple of the hospital blankets. Before you go, the nurse will show you how to use them to swaddle the baby. It looks easy! Fold, fold, tuck, fold, tuck, solve a differential equation, more tucking, and voilà!

When you get home and try it, you'll find it impossible to replicate. You can wrap up the baby, sure, but three minutes later, its arms are out and it's flailing around. You'll wonder, *Is it fold fold tuck, or fold tuck fold, or tuck fold fold tuck? Wait, was there something about an equation in there? Did I imagine that?*

Let me suggest you learn from the mistakes of those of us who have come before. If you want to swaddle, you cannot use a regular blanket. The nurses in the hospital can, but not you. Luckily, the market has solved this problem. There are a variety of blankets that will allow you to successfully swaddle your baby so they can't escape. The key is that these have some way of keeping your baby tucked in other than folding—for example, many yards of fabric or some Velcro. We used one called the Miracle Blanket.

Of course, you might ask, Why swaddle? Is there any reason to do this, or is it just adorable?

Swaddling is thought to improve sleep and decrease crying. If true, these are very good reasons to swaddle, since the main things babies seem to like to do are cry and not sleep. And fortunately, this turns out not to be very difficult to study, since sleep is a very short-term outcome. Researchers can look at the *same* baby swaddled and unswaddled. This avoids a lot of our concerns about different parents doing different things with their babies.

To give an example: One study followed twenty-six infants under three months of age.[2] The researchers brought the infants into a sleep lab, and observed them during both swaddled and unswaddled sleep. They used a special type of swaddle that could detect movement. It was basically a zippered bag, since even sleep researchers cannot fold successfully. In addition to the sensors, they also videotaped the babies to see what they were up to during sleep.

The study strongly supported the value of swaddling for sleep. While swaddled, the babies slept longer overall, with more time spent in REM sleep. This paper also identified the mechanism: swaddling improves sleep because it limits arousals.[3] Swaddled babies are equally likely to have the first stage in arousal—measured with baby "sighs"—but are less likely to move from this to the second stage ("startles") or the third ("fully awake"). Something about the swaddle discourages these second and third stages. These effects are big. The study found that when babies were not swaddled, a sigh turned into a startle 50 percent of the time. When they were swaddled, this occurred only 20 percent of the time. This type of laboratory evidence is confirmed by observational data and descriptive studies.

Swaddling may also limit crying, especially in newborns who are pre-term or have neurological issues. There are several small studies focused on infants with brain injuries or neonatal abstinence syndrome that have shown reductions in crying as a result of consistent swaddling.[4] Whether this translates to healthy infants who cry a lot is unclear, but certainly plausible.

There are some concerns about swaddling, and some cautions. First, in cultures where it is common to tightly swaddle infants all the time (for example, groups that tie babies to cradleboards), there is a risk of the in-fant developing hip dysplasia.[5] This is a condition where the hip bone is loose in the socket and can cause long-term pain and mobility difficulties if untreated. Although hip dysplasia can be treated with a harness or a body cast, it is not a trivial complication. These risks arise if the baby's legs are not able to flex at the hip, so it is crucial to swaddle the baby in a way that allows them to move their legs around. Most of the standard swaddle blankets are designed to allow this.

You'll also sometimes see swaddling discussed in connection with an increased risk of sudden infant death syndrome (SIDS). To the extent we have data, this concern does not seem valid, as long as you are putting the baby to sleep on its back (which you should do regardless).[6] Infants who are put to sleep on their stomach and are swaddled are at an increased risk of SIDS relative to those put to sleep on their stomach alone. But the crucial thing to avoid is putting your baby to sleep on their stomach, not swaddling.

Finally, some people worry that swaddling can lead to their infant overheating. This is possible in principle—if, say, you use a swaddle made from very heavy cloth and cover the baby's head in a hot room, especially if the child is sick—but it is not a significant risk in typical circumstances.

Obviously, you'll eventually have to take the kid out of the swaddle. Once they can roll over, you definitely want to have them out, since you do not want them on their stomach while swaddled. Even if you do not have a rolling kid, as the baby gets larger and stronger, they'll start fighting the swaddle, and you'll come into their room in the morning to find they have escaped, despite the blanket maker's assurance that this is impossible.

At this point, you pretty much have to cut it out, and are likely in for a few days of crying as the baby gets used to it. But as you know, Finn only fussed a bit when he lost his swaddle due to power outage. So I, personally, come down on the side of the swaddle.

COLIC AND CRYING

Most parents, especially with their first child, think their baby cries a lot. I certainly did. In the early months, Penelope had an especially sensitive period between five and eight p.m., during which she was often inconsolable. I'd walk her up and down the halls, bouncing up and down, sometimes just crying (me crying, that is—obviously she was crying). I once did this in a hotel—up and down, up and down, Penelope screaming at the top of her lungs. I hope no one else was staying there.

I remember this experience as exhausting—all those bouncing muscles—but also deeply frustrating. Why couldn't I get this to work? People had all kinds of suggestions. "Just nurse her!" (Attempts to do this made her cry more.) "Bounce faster." "Bounce slower." "Bounce more deeply." "No bouncing." "Swing while you bounce."

Both my mother and mother-in-law told me Jesse and I had been just the same. My mother-in-law, Joyce, said when she left the hospital with Jesse, the nurses said, "Good luck." So maybe it was genetic, or some kind of intergenerational payback.

By the time I had Penelope, I was thirty-one. Up to that point in my life, there had been surprisingly few instances in which I could not defeat a problem with hard work. General equilibrium theory comes to mind, but I had rarely found something where trying harder didn't make the problem at least somewhat better.

But you basically cannot defeat a crying baby with hard work. There may be some things that improve this in the moment, but babies cry— some of them cry a lot—and there is often really nothing you can do. In a sense, the most important thing to understand is that you are not alone and that your baby is not broken. How do we know you are not alone? That's what data is for.

Babies who cry a lot are often described as "colicky." Infantile colic isn't a biological diagnosis like strep throat, but a label we give to babies who cry a lot for no identifiable reason. A common definition of colic (although not the only one) is the rule of three: unexplained crying for more than three hours a day for more than three days a week for more than three weeks.

Based on this definition, colic is pretty rare. In one study of 3,300 babies, researchers found that at one month of age, 2.2 percent of babies fit the "rule of three" colic definition; this is similar at three months.[7] As you relax the definition, the shares go up. For example, if you look for babies who cry more than three hours a day for more than three days a week for more than one week (this is like the rule of 3-3-1), this share is 9 percent at one month. If you rely on parental reports that the infant "cries a lot," the share is close to 20 percent. This is probably not a good way to judge, but it gives a sense of how people experience infant crying.

Colic-type crying, whether it fits the rule of three exactly or not, is exhausting and depressing for new parents. Part of this definition is crying inconsolably—this isn't hungry crying or wet-diaper crying or tired crying. Infants will often arch their back, ball up their legs, and seem to be in distress or pain.

If you have an infant who cries a lot, whether it is true colic by the formal definition or not, the most important thing is to try to take care of yourself. Infant crying links to postpartum depression and anxiety, and parents—*both* parents—will need a break. Try to find one, even if it means leaving the infant crying in their crib for a few minutes while you shower. They will be fine. No, really, they will be fine. Take a shower. If you really cannot bear to leave them, call your best friend and tell them to come over and hold the crying baby. Call any random mom of an older kid, for that matter. They will do it.

It is also important to say that this is "self-limiting": colic will go away, typically around three months. Not all at once, but things will start to improve.

There are a few things that may improve colic, but since the cause of colic is poorly understood, solutions are hard to develop. Many of the theories involve digestion—poorly developed gut flora or an intolerance to milk protein. These are just theories, although, since they are the leading theories, most of the proposed solutions relate to them.

One commonly suggested solution, at least according to the internet, is simethicone, a gas-relieving drug (Gerber sells a set of these drops). There is no evidence to suggest this works. Trials are limited, and the two small trials that compared this treatment with a placebo showed no impact on crying. The same can be said of various herbal treatments and things like gripe water.[8]

Two treatments have some known success with colic. One is supplementation with a probiotic, which a number of studies have shown to reduce crying. These effects seem to show up only in breastfed infants.[9] This treatment isn't complicated—probiotics are delivered in drops, and Gerber and others make easily accessible over-the-counter versions. With no recognized downsides, probiotics are certainly worth a try.

The other treatment that has shown some success is managing the baby's diet, either by changing formula types or, if the baby is breastfed, changing the mother's diet. Changing formula is relatively straightforward, although the formulas appropriate for colic tend to be a bit more expensive. One recommendation is to switch to a soy-based or hydrolyzed protein formula[10] (most of the major formula makers—Similac, Enfamil—

have versions of these). The evidence on formula switching is mostly financed by formula companies, so do with that what you will, but it may be worth a try.

If you're breastfeeding, changing the baby's diet is complicated, since it means changing your own. There is some evidence supporting a "low-allergen" diet for Mom: randomized studies have shown reductions in crying and infant distress when mothers adopt this type of diet.[11] The standard recommendation is the elimination of all dairy, wheat, eggs, and nuts, so this means a pretty dramatic dietary change. Unfortunately, we don't know if just one of these foods, all, or a combination makes the difference, and the evidence is overall pretty limited (this definitely does not work for everyone).

The effects of this elimination diet seem to appear quickly if they appear at all—within the first few days of implementing the changes—so it is possible to try this and see if it works.[12] The obvious downside is that this change in diet is no fun at all for Mom and can make it hard to get enough calories, so there is some appropriate caution around making this a blanket recommendation. This is also likely not a time in your life when you're looking to experiment with new recipes. Still, without other options, there is reason to give it a try.

Regardless of what you do, your baby will still cry, sometimes for what seems to be no reason at all. It may not feel like it at the time, but this *will* go away, and you'll more or less forget about it as your child ages (this is presumably why people are willing to have a second child). Older babies do cry, but mostly for reasons you can understand or at least identify. Management of your own stress levels is at least as important as managing the baby's crying.

DATA COLLECTION

When we left the hospital with Penelope, the doctors and nurses suggested we keep track of how much she pooped and peed, since if an infant stops peeing, it is a sign of dehydration and needs to be monitored. This is good advice, and not that difficult to do.

What they did *not* suggest—but Jesse insisted we do anyway—was setting up a spreadsheet to enter this data. Jesse's idea was to keep track of everything that happened with Penelope in terms of feeding and diapers.

Here is day 4 of her life.

Date	Count per Day	Time	Left	Right	Dirty	Wet
4/12/2011	1	1:53:00	10	10	1	1
4/12/2011	2	3:50:00	20	10	1	1
4/12/2011	4	7:45:00		15	1	1
4/12/2011	5	10:00:00		10	1	1
4/12/2011	6	12:10:00	15	18		
4/12/2011	8	16:55:00	8	11	1	1
4/12/2011	9	17:55:00	15	6	1	1
4/12/2011	10	20:04:00	16	31	1	1

You'll notice that there are some more precise entries for breastfeeding times and some less so. The less precise entries are mine. Indeed, in some notes about this period that Jesse made for posterity, he indicated, "Dad set up a really elaborate data-entry system to log feeding and pooping. Mom wasn't really as good as Dad at keeping track of minutes. She liked to round to more even numbers."

Please remember, we are two economists married to each other. There is no hope for us.

At the two-week visit, we showed our spreadsheet to our pediatrician. She told us to cut it out.

Of course, we were amateurs at this relative to some other parents. My friends Hilary and John developed a complete statistical model, with graphs, of the relationship between eating and sleep length.

For people who love data, there is a seduction to seeing the numbers there in black and white. You can look for patterns—on one day, the baby slept for seven hours. Why was that? Was it the twenty-three minutes of nursing before? Should you try exactly that length of time again?

There are some (minimal) reasons to collect data. Keeping track of when the baby is eating can be valuable early on since it's easy to forget when they last ate. There are some nice apps that let you record from which breast they ate last. I know what you're thinking: *How could I forget that?* Trust me, you will. I used a system with a safety pin, which I moved from one side of my shirt to the other to tell me which breast to start with next. Not recommended; I frequently stabbed myself.

In the event that your infant is struggling to gain weight, keeping track of how often and how much they are eating (and, in some extreme cases, weighing them before and after feeding) can be very valuable. But for most babies, this is unlikely to be necessary or useful.

As the baby gets a bit older, keeping track of when the baby eats may help form a schedule. But in the first weeks, a feeding schedule is a bit of a pipe dream. If you want to collect data and make pretty graphs, go for it. But remember that this is the illusion of control, not actual control.

GERM EXPOSURE

There is a broad theory called the hygiene hypothesis, which states (I am paraphrasing here) that the increase in occurrences of allergies and other autoimmune illnesses over time is a result of decreased germ exposure in childhood, and that exposure to more microbes and germs as a child can help their immune system properly identify and not overreact to perceived pathogens.[13] While we don't have conclusive proof that this is true, there is some evidence backing the theory in the form of laboratory studies of particular cells and comparisons across cultures in rates of various diseases. This suggests that as your child ages—say, into toddlerhood and beyond—it is not necessarily a good idea to wipe down everything with hand sanitizer or bring your own disposable placemats to restaurants. Your kid probably shouldn't lick the floor at the airport, as mine have occasionally done, but going a bit more in the exposure direction may be sensible.

For these reasons, many doctors are reasonably lax about children's germ exposure after infancy. But virtually all doctors will suggest you try to avoid exposure to illness in the baby's first couple of months. One reason for this is simply that the smaller the child, the more vulnerable they are to serious complications. But a second reason is that for very young infants—especially those younger than twenty-eight days—medical protocols suggest much more aggressive interventions in response to illness.

What does this mean? Basically, if your otherwise well-seeming six-month-old gets a fever—even a pretty high one—and you go to the doctor, they'll probably look them over, tell you they have a virus, and send you home with instructions to give them Tylenol and fluids. In fact, many doctors' offices will tell you not to bring this child in at all unless you are very concerned.

In contrast, if your two-week-old has even a low fever, you'll need to take them to the hospital, where they'll be subjected to lab tests—likely including a lumbar puncture (spinal tap)—given antibiotics, and admitted as an inpatient. With very young babies, doctors have a harder time distinguishing between high- and low-risk fevers. Babies in this group are somewhat more susceptible to bacterial infections, including meningitis, which is extremely serious. Somewhere between 3 and 20 percent of infants under a month old who come to the doctor with a fever have a bacterial infection.[14] These are mostly urinary tract infections, but they must be treated, and reasonably quickly.

The combination of this higher risk of and difficulty detecting infection means that aggressive intervention is an appropriate approach, but most babies with fevers are actually fine.

When a slightly older infant—between twenty-eight days and two or three months—presents with a fever, there is more ambiguity about treatment. Some doctors will still perform a routine spinal tap, although there is less evidence that this is beneficial.[15] The procedure for managing infants in this age range (and younger) is many-stepped and varied.

Two of the key points here are whether the baby appears sick (this sounds crazy—of course they appear sick; they have a fever—but if you are a pediatrician, this distinction apparently makes sense) and whether there is an obvious viral exposure. If you come in with a forty-five-day-old baby who has a cold and a low-grade fever but seems otherwise fine, and bring along the baby's two-year-old sibling who has a cold from day care, the doctor is likely to react differently than if you come in with the same baby with no sibling, and the baby is listless.

How does this all relate to the question of germ exposure?

The big downside of being exposed to germs—or specifically, to sick kids—during these early weeks is the possibility of setting off this chain of interventions. If your infant does get sick, these procedures make sense, but if they just caught a cold from being pawed by a germy two-year-old, you'll be doing a lot of interventions for no reason. It's therefore better to keep the germy two-year-old away from the newborn, if at all possible.

Once your baby is over three months, and especially after they've had the first set of vaccines, treatment of a fever is closer to what you'd expect with an older child—basically, give them some Tylenol, keep them hydrated, and wait for it to go away. At this point, the downside of germ exposure is simply a sick kid, not a cascade of invasive testing.

The Bottom Line

- Swaddling has been shown to reduce crying and improve sleep. It is important to swaddle in a way that allows the baby to move its legs and hips.
- Colic is defined as excessive crying. *It is self-limiting*, meaning it will stop eventually. Changing formula or maternal diet, treatment with a probiotic, or both have shown some positive impacts.

continued . . .

- Collecting data on your baby is fun! But not necessary or especially useful.
- Exposing your infant to germs early on risks their getting sick, and the interventions for a feverish infant are aggressive and typically include a spinal tap. Limiting germ exposure may be a good idea, even if just to avoid these interventions.

3

Trust Me, Take the
Mesh Underwear

When I was pregnant with Penelope, Jesse and I went to a childbirth class at the hospital. Toward the end of the day, they handed around a bag of stuff that you'd be given after birth. There were ice packs and huge menstrual pads and these really enormous mesh underwear.

"These are the greatest!" enthused the person running the class. "You'll definitely want to take some home with you." I took a closer look. They were like parachutes. I mean, there is no question that my butt grew along with the rest of me, but would I seriously be wearing these? It was enough to make me reconsider the childbirth decision, but at that point it was a bit late.

It turns out that the mesh underwear—which, yes, you should take with you—is so large because it has to hold all the other stuff the hospital gives you. First you put on the underwear, then add a giant menstrual pad or four, and finally a layer of ice packs. It's a makeshift ice diaper.

There are a lot of baby books (like this one) that tell you what will happen with your baby. And there are a lot of pregnancy books that detail what happens to you while you are pregnant. But the world is oddly lacking in discussions of what happens, physically, to Mom after the baby arrives. Before the baby, you're a vessel to be cherished and protected. After the baby, you're a lactation-oriented baby accessory.

This omission is problematic, since it fails to inform women about what to expect *after* you're expecting. Physical recovery from childbirth is not always straightforward, and even in the best of circumstances, it's messy. Hence, the ice diaper.

In this chapter, I talk a bit about what you can expect for your body in the first days and weeks after you've given birth. I should clarify that the discussion here covers a typical recovery. Things can go wrong in ways beyond this, which is why it is crucial to tell your doctor if you are concerned about anything. The lack of discussion of what to expect in terms of your post-childbirth body can make it seem like anything you're experiencing is fine, but it's not. There is no shame in asking.

(I should add a caution here, for which you can thank my friend Tricia: if you have already been through this and you do not want to relive the gory details, skip to the next chapter.)

IN THE DELIVERY ROOM

The baby has arrived. The delivery is over. The placenta is out. If the birth—either vaginal or by caesarean section—went as expected, they'll likely let you hold the baby and perhaps encourage you to try to nurse.

In the meantime, the doctor will be working on repairing things.

If you've had a caesarean, your doctor will stitch up the incision and dress the wound. This is typically a straightforward process, and similar from woman to woman. With a vaginal birth, there is more variation. During a vaginal birth it is very common to have vaginal tearing. This most frequently involves the perineum—the area between the vagina and anus—but you can also have tearing in the direction of the clitoris.

The degree of this tearing varies widely across women. Some women do not tear (although most women do a bit, at least with their first baby). If you do tear, the degree is ranked from first to fourth degree. A first-degree laceration is minor tearing, which heals well on its own with no stitches. Second degree means there is more involvement of the perineal muscles, but the tear doesn't extend to the anus. Third- and fourth-degree tears extend all the way from the vagina to the anus but differ in how deep they go, with fourth-degree tears extending into the rectum. Third- and fourth-degree tears must be repaired with stitches, which will dissolve on their own after a few weeks.

Most tears are on the minor side, but approximately 1 to 5 percent of women will have more serious third- and fourth-degree tears.[1] More severe tearing is more common with instrument-assisted delivery (that is, delivery with either forceps or a vacuum). There is some evidence that warm compresses on the perineum during the pushing stage of labor can prevent very severe tears.

Depending on the degree of tearing, the repair can take quite a while. If you've had an epidural, you should not feel the stitching. If you did not have an epidural, it's common for the doctor to use a local anesthetic.

The other thing that will happen in the delivery room and continue over the next few hours is abdominal massage. Over the first hours after birth, the uterus should contract toward its pre-pregnancy size. If this doesn't happen, there is an increased risk of bleeding. Uterine, or "fundal," massage has been shown to assist this process and lower the risk of bleeding. A strong nurse will come around occasionally and push hard on your stomach. This is uncomfortable at a minimum. (To call this a "massage" is an insult to even the worst massage therapist.) With Finn, the nurse who did this told me, "I'm not the nurse people like to see." If you've had a caesarean, it can be extremely painful. The good news is that you shouldn't need abdominal massage after the first twelve to twenty-four hours.

IN THE RECOVERY ROOM
AND BEYOND

When things are fixed up, you'll head off to the recovery room to begin trying to get back to normal (except now you have a baby). Of course, you're not quite the old you.

Bleeding

Regardless of how you gave birth, for the first couple of days afterward, you will bleed *a lot*. Before I had Penelope, I was under the impression that this bleeding was due to trauma; this isn't the case (or, at least, you will bleed even without trauma). In fact, it is the lining of the uterus departing.

For the first day or two, this bleeding—in particular, the clotted blood—can be a little scary. You'll sit down to pee or get up out of the bed and there will be an enormous blood clot in the toilet or on the pad. The doctors will tell you to watch out for clots "fist size or larger" (other doctors will use fruit metaphors—a plum- or small orange–size clot, they want to know about). By extension, this means that clots smaller than that—but not much smaller—are common. Passing these isn't typically painful, but it is jarring.

You can bleed too much—maternal hemorrhage is a possible postbirth complication. Since you know you should bleed some, it can be hard to know how much is too much. If you're not sure, ask. If you see a clot and think, *Is that the size of a fist, or just a bit smaller?*, don't wait around measuring it for yourself—buzz the nurse.

The passing of clots will die down after a couple of days, but you'll keep bleeding—first like a heavy period, then a lighter period—for weeks. Once you're home, the bleeding should decrease over time. If, all of a sudden, you start bleeding a lot again, especially if the blood is bright red, call your doctor immediately.

Peeing and Pooping

Many women get a catheter (a tube in the urethra to collect pee) during birth—you'll get this for sure if you have a caesarean, and very likely if you have an epidural. This will be removed in the first few hours afterward, and it will be time to try to pee and poop on your own.

The experience here begins to diverge depending on what kind of birth you had.

If you had a vaginal birth, it will hurt to pee. Even if you had a very "easy" experience, your vagina will still be kind of banged up, and there will be some stinging. It's worse if you are dehydrated, which makes the urine more concentrated. At many hospitals, they'll give you a squeeze bottle of water, the idea being that you squeeze water on *while* you pee so the urine is diluted and not as painful. This works okay, although—here's a pro tip—definitely make sure you do not use extremely cold water.

It will also likely hurt to poop. This depends, again, on how traumatic your birth experience was. It is common to give women stool softeners to improve the first postbirth bowel movement. It may be a couple of days before you actually have that first bowel movement, which is good. Also, this may not be as bad as you think. And anyway, you have to do it.

If you have had a caesarean, these problems are different. First, you may struggle with holding pee at all while you wait for your bladder to "wake up" after surgery, and the catheter may be left in place longer. Whether peeing will hurt depends on the circumstances of your labor and delivery. If you were in labor for a long time before the surgery, you may still have discomfort and swelling that makes urination uncomfortable. With a scheduled C-section, this may not happen.

After a caesarean, doctors generally want you to either poop or at least pass some gas before you leave the hospital; this is to ensure that you can have a bowel movement after what is basically major abdominal surgery. It is not unusual for it to take several days for this to happen. In service of this, you'll get stool softeners. In the absence of vaginal trauma, the actual act may not be that uncomfortable. Sitting down, however, can be painful due to your incision.

Lingering Consequences

A few days later, you're home. The most immediate consequences—heavy bleeding, uncomfortable first pee, etc.—will be over.

You will not, however, feel normal.

First of all, you'll still look pregnant. This appearance will subsist for a few days or weeks. Then you'll just have a bunch of floppy skin. This does resolve eventually (by which I mean weeks or months later, not days), but it's a little disconcerting to look down at. Even once the floppy skin is gone, many of us find we have what is referred to as "mummy tummy," a pouchy stomach that doesn't ever seem to quite snap back. I can find no literature on this, but I assure you it is a real thing that no amount of Pilates can get rid of (and by "no amount" I specifically mean one hour a week with Larry, whose other clients are mostly elderly women).

If you had a vaginal birth, the most significant lingering physical consequences are for your vagina. As one medical description puts it, "After birth, the vagina will be capacious."[2]

Things will just not be quite the way they were before. You may have stitches; the whole area will be painful and just kind of off. It is not the vagina you are familiar with.

This does heal, but it takes time, and for most women, things don't quite go back to the way they were before birth. (This doesn't necessarily mean worse, just different.) And your vagina will definitely not be back to normal two weeks later. The rest of you might be feeling pretty normal at this point (minus the pudgy tummy, the exhaustion, and the enormous boobs), but this could also take longer—it took you forty weeks to stretch out, so it's hard to rush going back.

With a caesarean section, your problems will be different. Depending on how it went down, you may have little or no vaginal trauma. As one friend with a scheduled C-section told me, "No one got anywhere near my vagina." Not everyone is so lucky—if you got far into labor before needing surgery, you'll have a recovery not dissimilar from a woman who's had a vaginal birth. And every C-section, planned or not, is major abdominal surgery, meaning it will be painful to do anything that involves your abdominal muscles. This includes walking, going up stairs, sitting, picking things up, rolling over, etc. Everything you do just hurts.

Here's an example: Say you're in bed and you're thirsty in the middle of the night. Your painkillers have worn off and you reach for your water. This is extremely painful.

The pain and discomfort will get better over time, but (on average) it will take longer to feel like you're back to normal than if you'd had a vaginal birth.

Regardless of how you gave birth, it's a good idea to have help, but this is especially important if you've had a caesarean. You need someone around who can help you get up, get to the bathroom, do the activities of daily life. Even if you can handle the baby on your own, someone needs to help handle you. Depending on your recovery, it may be a challenge to even lift the baby on your own for the first week or two. With a complicated caesarean (or even a complicated vaginal birth), it might be weeks before you feel like you can get up and shower alone.

With both vaginal and caesarean deliveries, there are other common, mostly minor, lingering consequences. Hemorrhoids, for example. Also, incontinence. Many women find that after childbirth, they pee a bit when they cough or laugh, or seemingly for no reason. This, like other things, will improve over time.

Women will have a wide range of experiences during recovery, regardless of how they gave birth. I had a very lucky draw with both my children. With Finn, I walked out of the hospital twelve hours later, carrying his car seat. But this isn't the norm, and even then it wasn't as if I was running a marathon anytime soon (or ever). Much of what determines your experience is luck, or some anatomy of your pelvis. Perhaps the most important thing is to ask for help when you need it, and not to expect so much. Many cultures have a tradition of women basically doing nothing for a month or so after birth, while older women in their family take care of them. This isn't common in the US, but it does give a sense of what this time is like. Just because some fit-pregnancy blogger is back to CrossFit ten days after giving birth does not mean her recovery is typical.

Serious Complications

Post-delivery, some rare, serious complications can arise. These include excessive bleeding, dangerously high blood pressure, and infection. Risks vary across women—infection, for example, is a more common risk for women who have had a caesarean. Your doctor will likely tell you what to look out for, based on your own birth experience and any particular complications from it.

There are a few specific red flags to look out for:

- Fever
- Severe abdominal pain
- Increase in bleeding, especially bright red blood
- Bad-smelling vaginal discharge
- Chest pain or shortness of breath

In addition, it is important to pay attention to any changes in vision, serious headaches, or increasing swelling (say, in your ankles), especially if you had or were at risk for preeclampsia.

These instructions can be hard to remember in the haze of new parenting, though. If something doesn't seem quite right to you, call your doctor.

EXERCISE AND SEX

While you are struggling to roll over in bed for a drink of water, dealing with the world's heaviest period, and also caring for someone who cries all the time, exercise and sex may not be your first priorities. On the other hand, exercise and sex were likely among your pre-birth activities, and in an effort to return to feeling like yourself, you may want to get back to them.

So despite the barriers, many of us do wonder, *When is it okay to get back on the treadmill, or back in bed?*

In the case of exercise, there is relatively little concrete evidence on when it is okay to start. The American College of Obstetricians and Gynecologists says that it is safe to resume exercise "within a few days" after a normal vaginal delivery. This isn't to say you will be running interval workouts a week later, but some walking may be feasible.

They caution, though, that this will be different if you've had a caesarean or significant vaginal tearing. In the case of a caesarean, the standard recommendations include some walking within the first two weeks, introducing the possibility of abdominal curls or other related exercises by week 3 and a resumption of "normal" activities by around week 6.[3] Again, healing rates differ from woman to woman, so this is really just an average.

In the case of vaginal delivery, where the issue is tearing, return to exercise should be even faster, with appropriate care taken to make sure you feel okay. Nearly all people—including elite athletes, but also recreational athletes and those of us who just walk or run for exercise—should be able to resume pre-pregnancy activity levels by six weeks postpartum and some modified version before that.

If you are an elite athlete, even a couple of weeks may seem like a long period to be off training, and depending on circumstances, it may be possible to work with your doctor to more quickly get back to training. But honestly, outside this group, the physical ability to exercise will probably arrive substantially before you are mentally ready to take advantage of it.

Once you can exercise, it can be challenging to find time in your schedule, but if it's important to you, you should try. Exercise can help combat postpartum depression and generally improves mood. Yes, there are other demands on your time, but taking care of yourself also matters.

When it comes to sex after baby, there is a commonly accepted rule: no sex until six weeks postpartum, after you have had a checkup with your doctor. This is so often cited that I had assumed it was evidence based, that there was some biological reason why you need to wait this long, no more, no less.

In fact, this is completely fabricated. There is no set waiting period for resuming sex after giving birth. The six-week rule appears to have been invented by doctors so husbands wouldn't ask for sex. This somewhat odd tradition persists. When I had my first postpartum checkup around six weeks after having Finn, the doctor (not my midwife, but the doctor who happened to be available that day) told me I was fine, and then asked if I wanted him to write me a note to tell my husband I was not. I found this very uncomfortable.

This is not to say there are no real guidelines for when you can resume having sex. Physically, if you have had tearing, it is important to wait until the perineum is healed. Depending on the severity of the tearing, this could happen much before six weeks, or it could take longer. Your doctor will check this at your first postpartum checkup (which is, in fact, around six weeks), but you may be able to tell if you've healed before that.

There are two other considerations. First, contraception: Even if you are breastfeeding and just had a baby three weeks ago, you can get pregnant. Most people do not plan babies ten months apart, so unless you have, make sure you are using some kind of birth control. (And think carefully about what type: some kinds of birth control, specifically some birth control pills, can interfere with milk production.)

The other consideration is, as the medical guidelines state, "emotional readiness." You need to *want* to have sex. There is a tremendous amount of variation across women (and their partners) in when they feel ready to resume sex after giving birth. And you both need to be ready.

Birth is a very physical ordeal—even with a pretty easy birth, there will be physical consequences for at least a few weeks. Also, three or four weeks in, your family is likely to be exhausted. The baby may still be eating every two or three hours, and the idea of spending some of the time between feedings having sex, as opposed to sleeping or showering or eating, may seem laughable.

This is, of course, the standard story. But it is probably important to say that some people *do* want to have sex a few weeks later—and not just the non-birthing parents, either. If you are healed up and you want to have sex, go for it.

Looking at the data—which, in this case, may not be so helpful, since really the question is when *you* want to do it—most couples have resumed at least some sexual activity by eight weeks postpartum. For those with an uncomplicated vaginal delivery, the average is about five weeks, versus six weeks for caesarean and seven for those with significant vaginal tearing.[4] Having said this, it takes an average of about a year to get back to pre-pregnancy sex frequency, and many people never return to having quite as much sex as they did before.

A final note: Sex after childbirth can be painful. Breastfeeding promotes vaginal dryness and lowers your sex drive. In addition, injuries during birth can have persistent effects. Many women, after having a small person attached to them nearly constantly, really do not want to be touched. Most women need some lubrication the first few times they have sex after giving birth to deal with vaginal dryness. And you want to take it slow at the start. And, of course, this all focuses on penetrative vaginal sex. Other activities—oral sex, either given or received—may be easier to restart, and could be more enjoyable early on.

Many women experience continued pain and discomfort during sex long after giving birth. This is not something you should ignore or grit your teeth and learn to live with. There are treatments that can help, including physical therapy. If sex is painful, talk to your doctor about it. If they're not comfortable discussing it, find a doctor who is.

EMOTIONAL HEALTH: POSTPARTUM DEPRESSION, ANXIETY, AND PSYCHOSIS

So far, this discussion has dealt with the physical consequences of childbirth. But there are also often serious emotional consequences. Postpartum depression, postpartum anxiety, and even postpartum psychosis are common, to varying degrees. Too many women suffer from these conditions in silence, and this needs to stop.

In the first days and weeks after your baby arrives, you will experience a wave of hormones. Most women find they are emotionally sensitive during this period. This is not, for example, the time to watch the first fifteen minutes of the movie *Up*.

In thinking about this period, I recall our first outing, to a brunch at a friend's house when Penelope was a week old. I spent two hours hiding in their guest room, nursing and crying. There wasn't anything wrong; I just couldn't stop crying. It was set off, I think, by the realization that the hat I had carefully knitted for Penelope was too large. And that once she did fit into it, it would probably be too warm to wear it. This was enough to sustain several hours of tears.

I'm lucky these were good friends, who brought me brunch on a tray. Of course, that only made me cry more.

This early experience is sometimes referred to as the "baby blues" and is self-limiting in the sense that the hormone surge is worst in the first few days after giving birth and dies down a couple of weeks later.

But true postpartum depression or other postpartum mental health conditions can crop up in this period. They can also arise later, even months later. Many women discount later-onset depression, thinking postpartum depression happens only right after the baby arrives. This is not the case.

The prevalence of postpartum depression, even if we focus only on diagnosed cases, is high. An estimated 10 to 15 percent of women who give birth will experience it.[5] Most obstetricians are trained to look for depression during pregnancy, but, although less acknowledged, the data suggests that about half of these women actually experience the onset of depression *during* pregnancy, something many people are surprised to learn. Women are otherwise typically (although not exclusively) diagnosed with postpartum depression within the first four months.

There are some important risk factors for postpartum depression. These fall into two categories: predisposition and situation. By far the biggest risk factor for postpartum depression is predisposition, or prior experience of depression. Mental health isn't as well understood as we would like, but there are clearly some genetic or epigenetic factors that affect it. If you've had episodes of depression before, they are more likely to crop up again in pregnancy or in the postpartum period. Be on the lookout for signs, and get help if you see them.

The other risk factors are largely about situation. Some of these factors are modifiable, some are not. Women (or men) who have less social support, who experience difficult life events around this time, or whose baby has medical or other problems are more likely to be depressed. And the baby itself can also play a role; people with babies who are poor sleepers are at greater risk for depression, almost certainly due to the fact that they, in turn, get less sleep.

How is postpartum depression diagnosed? Ideally, every woman is screened for this using a short questionnaire at their six-week postpartum visit. The most widely used questionnaire is probably the Edinburgh Postnatal Depression Scale, though a few others are common. Here it is:

EDINBURGH POSTNATAL DEPRESSION SCALE

In the past 7 days:

1. I have been able to laugh and see the funny side of things.

❑ Yes, all the time	❑ Yes, most of the time	❑ No, not very often	❑ No, never

2. I have looked forward with enjoyment to things.

❑ As much as I always could	❑ Not quite so much now	❑ Definitely not so much now	❑ Not at all

3. I have blamed myself unnecessarily when things went wrong.

❑ Yes, most of the time	❑ Yes, some of the time	❑ Not very often	❑ No, never

4. I have been anxious or worried for no good reason.

❑ Not, not at all	❑ Hardly ever	❑ Yes, some-times	❑ Yes, very often

5. I have felt scared or panicky for no good reason.

❑ Yes, quite a lot	❑ Yes, some-times	❑ No, not much	❑ No, not at all

6. Things have been getting on top of me.

❑ Yes, most of the time I haven't been able to cope at all	❑ Yes, some-times I haven't been coping as well as usual	❑ No, most of the time I have coped quite well	❑ No, I have been coping as well as ever

7. I have been so unhappy that I have difficulty sleeping.

❑ Yes, most of the time	❑ Yes, sometimes	❑ Not very often	❑ No, not at all

8. I have felt sad or miserable.

❑ Yes, most of the time	❑ Yes, quite often	❑ Not very often	❑ No, not at all

9. I have been so unhappy that I have been crying.

❑ Yes, most of the time	❑ Yes, quite often	❑ Only occasionally	❑ No, never

10. The thought of harming myself has occurred to me.

❑ Yes, quite often	❑ Sometimes	❑ Hardly ever	❑ Never

The scaling of this is simple: Each answer is scored from 0 to 3, with the worst category (the first one for most questions, the last for 1, 2, and 4) getting a 3. Doctors will typically use a cutoff of 10 or 12 as a signal of mild depression, and a value of 20 or more as signaling a more serious depression.

Some of the questions here seem so obvious that it can be hard to imagine you'd actually need a questionnaire—can't you just ask people if they feel sad and disengaged? But the evidence suggests that using this screening tool can be extremely effective. Researchers have shown improvements in detection (and therefore treatment) of postpartum depression across a large number of women by using this questionnaire—as much as a 60 percent reduction in depression a few months later.[6] Your doctor will certainly give you this at your postpartum visit, but it isn't a bad idea to do some self-screening also, which could capture your prevailing mood better.

Treatment for postpartum depression proceeds in stages. For mild depression, the first line of treatment is to try to treat without drugs. There is some evidence that exercise or massage can be helpful. Or, perhaps most important, sleep. For new parents, in particular, lack of sleep can be a huge contributor to mild depression. This shouldn't be that surprising. Even when you don't have an infant, if you have a few nights of poor sleep, it can be hard to enjoy things. Now add together many, many nights of interrupted sleep—it's not surprising this could contribute to emotional exhaustion and depression.

Obviously, it is hard to treat lack of sleep when you have a newborn, although when I discuss sleep training later in the book, one of the strong arguments in favor of it is that it alleviates maternal depression. If you haven't sleep trained your baby, or don't plan to, or your baby is too young, there are still ways to improve your sleep. Get help for a night or two—or more—from a grandparent or friend. Hire a nighttime doula if possible. Divide the night duties with your partner so you can each get at least one uninterrupted stretch of sleep. It may be helpful to remind yourself that addressing your depression is valuable for your baby, too, not just some kind of selfish personal indulgence.

Beyond sleep, some type of cognitive behavioral therapy, or other talk therapy, is a usual first-line treatment for many people. This focuses on reframing negative thoughts and focusing on positive actions.

For more severe depression—sometimes defined as a score above 20 on the standard depression screen—antidepressants are more widely used. Although antidepressants are passed through breast milk, there is no evidence of adverse consequences (more on this in chapter 5). This means there is no need to choose between getting the help you need and nursing your baby.

Much of the literature and popular discourse focus on postpartum depression. But not all postpartum mental health issues take the form of depression. Postpartum anxiety is also common. Many of the symptoms are similar to postpartum depression, and indeed, it is common to diagnose postpartum anxiety using the same screening tool. But women with postpartum anxiety also tend to find themselves fixated on terrible things that could happen to the baby, unable to sleep even if the opportunity is there, and engaging in obsessive-compulsive behaviors around infant safety. This can be treated with therapy or, in more severe cases, with medication.

With anxiety, it can be hard to know where the line is between normal parental worry and obsessive worry. If anxiety is interfering with your ability to enjoy spending time with your baby, if it is occupying all your thoughts and preventing you from sleeping—that is over the line.

Less common but much more severe is postpartum psychosis.[7] This affects an estimated 1 to 2 in 1,000 women (versus 1 in 10 for postpartum depression) and is much more likely to develop in women with a history of bipolar disorder. Postpartum psychosis usually manifests in hallucinations, delusions, and manic episodes. It will very likely need inpatient treatment, and should be taken extremely seriously.

Although women who give birth are at greater risk of these mental health complications due to some combination of hormones and often being the primary caregiver, postpartum depression can crop up in non-birth parents, too. Dads, other moms, adoptive parents—all can experience these symptoms. And because screening is so often focused only on women who have given birth and not on others in the household, these diagnoses are missed much more frequently.

It wouldn't be a bad idea to have every adult in the household do a depression screen a few weeks after the baby is born, and then periodically after that. But if you are worried, call your doctor. Don't wait to see them at six weeks; the sooner you can get on top of these issues, the sooner you'll be able to enjoy your time with your baby, and the better things will be for everyone.

There are many issues in the pre-pregnancy, pregnancy, and post-pregnancy world that we do not talk about enough. When I was writing about pregnancy, the thing that struck me in this category was miscarriage. So many women have had miscarriages, yet they are rarely talked about—until you have one and then it turns out many women you know have also miscarried.

Postpartum mental and physical health have the same pattern. You have a new baby—shouldn't you be happy and feeling great? When people ask how you are, everyone wants to hear "The baby is great! We're so thrilled!" Not "I'm depressed and anxious and I'm dealing with third-degree vaginal tears." The fact that these things are not talked about makes many of us feel like we are the only ones dealing with them, or should just get over it.

This simply isn't true, and I think the more we talk about this, the more we do a service to other women. I'm not suggesting we all start tweeting the details of our vaginal healing—although I have no problem with that—but it is time to have a more honest conversation about the post-childbirth physical and mental experiences.

The Bottom Line

- It takes time to recover from childbirth.
  - You'll bleed for several weeks.
  - You may have vaginal tearing, which takes a few weeks to heal.
  - A caesarean section is major abdominal surgery, and it will take significant time for you to be mobile again afterward.
- Return to exercise depends a bit on your birth experience, but you can typically start within a week or two, and most women could be back to their pre-pregnancy routine by six weeks.
- There is no set waiting time for sex, although you should wait until you're ready (and are on birth control if you're not ready for another child).
- Postpartum depression (and related conditions) are common and treatable. Get help as soon as you need it.

PART TWO

The First Year

B reastfeeding. Sleep training. Co-sleeping. Vaccination. To work or not to work. Day care versus nanny.

These are the big decisions that will shape at least the first year of your life as a parent. They are decisions that, up until you became a parent, you probably never thought about. And the answers are not obvious.

So we turn to the internet. Which is great, since people on the internet have the answer. In fact, it's an answer that is easy to summarize and understand. The correct decision, in all cases, is to do exactly whatever that particular person on the internet did. More than that, making any other choice is roughly equivalent to abandoning your child to wolves.

Welcome to the Mommy Wars. So pleased you could join us.

Why are these particular topics so fraught? Why does it feel like an all-or-nothing battle? Why are these the focal points for our parenting anxiety and judgment?

I'm not sure, but I suspect it relates to the fact that the choices you make in these areas will dramatically affect your parenting experience. Whether you choose to breastfeed, whether you choose to have your child sleep in your room (or in your bed), whether you sleep train—you'll experience these choices every day.

And many of these choices make your life more difficult, or at least more annoying. Breastfeeding has some wonderful moments, but among the hundreds of women I have talked to about it, not one has told me,

"Lugging around the pumping parts everywhere was a fulfilling experience of womanhood!" Getting up four times a night until your child is one (or two, or two and a half . . .) is exhausting. It affects your mood, your work, your relationships.

At the same time, choosing to not breastfeed, or choosing to let your kid cry themselves to sleep a few times, is hard in a different way. People will judge you for these decisions, and, if we are being honest, you may judge yourself. Letting your kid cry themselves to sleep does work: most kids (and, thus, their parents) will sleep better afterward. Are you just being selfish and sacrificing your children's well-being for your own?

This is a good time to reiterate what I said in the introduction: like all other things in parenting, there is no perfect set of choices for everyone. There is a right set of choices for you, taking into account your preferences and your constraints. If you have six months off from work or are not going back to work at all, it may be easier to sacrifice sleep at night in exchange for napping during the day. If you work in an office with an opaque door where you can pump and work at the same time, it might be easier to nurse longer than if you have to sign up for time in the lactation pod (or, god forbid, the bathroom) and stop working to pump.

The fact that preferences matter, however, doesn't mean there's no room for facts. We cannot hope to make the right choices for ourselves without seeing the data. You and I may see the same data and make different decisions, but we should both come to the data as the first step. As an economist, I try to start my decisions with the data—What does it say? How confident are we in its findings?—and then try to think about what works for my family in light of that data. It helps to be married to another economist, but I'd argue that the language of data and preferences can work for anyone. You do not have to pay the costs of the two-economist marriage to reap the benefits.

This part of the book goes through the data on these major early parenting decisions. In many cases, the work of the book is really to separate the good studies on these topics from the less-good ones. In making decisions, we want to know the *causal* effect of one variable on another, not just that they are associated. It is no good to tell you that a kid who was breastfed differs from one who wasn't; you want to know whether the breastfeeding itself matters.

How can you identify a good study? This is a hard question. Some things you can see directly. Certain approaches are better than others—randomized trials, for example, are usually more compelling than other designs. Larger studies tend, on average, to be better. More studies confirming the same thing tends to increase confidence, although not always—sometimes they all have the same biases in their results.

I read a lot of studies—for this book, but also for my job—so some of my conclusions come from experience. Sometimes you poke into a study and it doesn't smell quite right—the groups they are comparing are really different, or the way they measure variables is skewed. Sometimes there will be a really big study, but it will be deeply flawed, and I'll end up relying more on a smaller study that has a better design.

And, sadly, for those of us who love data, the data will never be perfect.

In confronting the questions here, we also have to confront the limits of the data and the limits of *all* data. There are no perfect studies, so there will always be some uncertainty about conclusions. Beyond that, in many cases the only data we have is problematic—there will be a single, not-very-good study, and all we can say is that one study really doesn't support a relationship.

This means we can't ever say for sure that we're *certain* something is good or not good for a baby. Of course, sometimes we are more sure than others, and I'll try to let you know when the data really helps us see a relationship as true, and when there just isn't much for us to go on.

I hope you'll leave this section armed with some facts. Facts about what we know, but also facts about what we still don't know—places where the data is just uncertain, or hasn't provided a compelling answer. Armed with these facts, you can go forward to make your choices. Not the same choices, mind you. But the right ones for you.

Breast Is Best? Breast Is Better?
Breast Is About the Same?

The hospital at which I delivered Penelope had a lot of pre-delivery classes, one of which was about breastfeeding. I asked a friend with a slightly older baby if I should take it; she scrunched up her face and said, "You know, it's really not the same with a doll."

Boy, was that right. I am going to tell you the truth. For many women, including myself, breastfeeding was hard. (This doesn't mean the classes aren't useful, just that they aren't a panacea.)

When Penelope lost weight in the hospital, we had to supplement with formula. This might have been unnecessary. But what seemed even crazier was the very elaborate setup the nurse suggested for avoiding the dreaded "nipple confusion."

Rather than just handing me a bottle and suggesting I try that, I found myself hooked up to a system in which a tube was taped to my breast and the formula bottle was held above my head. We tried to nurse that way, with the formula being delivered through the tube, but neither Penelope nor I had any idea what we were doing.

They offered to send this system home with us, but I declined; if we needed to feed Penelope formula, it was going to come from a bottle.

My milk did eventually come in, but that wasn't the end of it. Much of the time, it still seemed like I didn't have enough. Before going to sleep at night, Penelope would eat and eat and eat, mostly from the bottle. I felt terrible. Everyone said, "Oh, if she still seems hungry, just let her keep trying to nurse. Your supply will catch up!" But she was clearly starving (at least, that's what it seemed like).

At the same time, I was trying to pump, to increase my supply and to have some backup for when I went back to work. But when to do this? Should I pump right after feeding her? What if she needed to eat again? Should I pump an hour after feeding her while she was napping? What if she woke up right after I finished and needed to eat again?

And worst, Penelope seemed to hate breastfeeding, and getting her to latch on was a struggle every time. When she was seven weeks old, we went to my brother's wedding, and I remember sitting in a back closet at the restaurant, where it was approximately one billion degrees, trying desperately to get her to latch on as she screamed and screamed. Eventually, we left the closet and I fed her a bottle in the air conditioning.

Why did I continue? With hindsight, I have no idea. Eventually, around three months, she finally just seemed to accept that I was not giving up and just started nursing one day without a lot of objections.

Breastfeeding isn't always like this, even from one baby to the next. With Finn, nursing was a breeze (other things were complicated). My milk came in faster, there was more of it, and he never had trouble figuring it out. And for some people, it's like this the first time.

But any struggle we experience is made worse by the emphasis— societal, familial, personal—on the many benefits of breastfeeding.

Here, for example, is a list of the *claimed* benefits of breastfeeding, which I pulled from a couple of websites.[1] (I should note that this chapter is focused on the benefits of breastfeeding in the US or other developed countries, where the formula alternative is safe and can be made with clean water. In developing countries, breastfeeding benefits are larger and different, since the alternative is often formula made with contaminated water.)

The list is very long, so I've divided it into sections.

Short-Term Baby Benefits	Long-Term Child Benefits: Health	Long-Term Child Benefits: Cognitive	Benefits for Mom	Benefits for the World
• Fewer colds, infections • Fewer allergic rashes • Fewer gastro-intestinal disorders • Lower risk of NEC • Lower risk of SIDS	• Less diabetes • Less juvenile arthritis • Lower risk of childhood cancer • Lower risk of meningitis • Lower risk of pneumonia • Lower risk of urinary tract infections • Lower risk of Crohn's disease • Lower risk of obesity • Lower risk of allergies, asthma	• Higher IQ	• Free birth control • More weight loss • Better bonding with your baby • Save money • More stress resistant • More sleep • Form better friendships • Lower risk of cancer • Lower risk of osteoporosis • Lower risk of postpartum depression	• Lower methane produc-tion from cows

You will note that one of these benefits is "better friendships." Really? Don't get me wrong—it can be lonely and isolating to be a new mom, and meeting other moms is a great idea. That's what stroller yoga is for. But I'm hard-pressed to figure out which of my friendships were enhanced by my attempts to feed a screaming baby in a hot closet.

And it is true that I can find no peer-reviewed evidence—reliable or otherwise—to suggest that friendships are enhanced by breastfeeding. Many of the benefits cited here do, however, have some basis in evidence, just not always especially *good* evidence.

In particular, as I mentioned in the introduction, most studies of breast-feeding are biased by the fact that women who breastfeed are typically different from those who do not. In the US, and most developed countries, more educated and richer women are more likely to nurse their babies.

This wasn't always the case. Breastfeeding has come in and out of fashion over the years, including over the past century. In the early part of the twentieth century, nearly all women breastfed, if they were physically able to, but the introduction of more "modern" formula starting around the 1930s led to a rapid decline in breastfeeding. This is likely, at least in part, because breastfeeding has always been hard. By the 1970s, the majority of women fed their babies with formula. But public health campaigns beginning at that time promoted the benefits of breastfeeding, pushing back against the trend of using formula. In response to this changed climate, formula manufacturers themselves did some breastfeeding promotion. Breastfeeding rates have increased since then. This increase has been greater in some groups than others, notably among more educated and richer women.[2]

The relationship between breastfeeding and education, income, and other variables is a problem for research. Having more education and more resources is linked to better outcomes for infants and children, even independent of breastfeeding. This makes it very difficult to infer the *causal* effect of breastfeeding. Sure, there is a correlation between nursing and various good outcomes—but that doesn't mean that for an individual woman, nursing her baby will make the child better off.

To give a concrete example, take one study, conducted in the late 1980s, of 345 Scandinavian children that compared IQ scores at age five for children who were breastfed for less than three months versus more than six months.[3] The authors found that the children who nursed longer had higher IQ scores—about a seven-point difference. But the mothers who breastfed longer were also richer, had more education, and had higher IQ scores themselves. Once the authors adjusted for even a few of these variables, the effects of nursing were much, much smaller.

The authors of this and other studies claim that once they adjust for the differences they see across women, the effects persist. But this assumes that the adjustments they make are able to remove *all* the differences across women, and this is extremely unlikely.

For example, in most studies of breastfeeding, researchers do not have access to the mother's IQ. More commonly, they'll see a measure of the mother's education, which is related to IQ. On average, a woman with a college degree will perform better on an IQ test than a woman with less than a high school degree. But these education categories are not a fully accurate measure of IQ.

When we look at breastfeeding, we find that mothers with higher IQ scores are more likely to nurse their babies, even within groups of mothers of the same education level.[4] Those mothers with higher IQs, again among peers of the same education level, also have (on average) children with higher IQs.[5] Even if researchers are able to adjust for a mother's education, they are still left with a situation in which breastfeeding behavior is associated with other characteristics (in this example, maternal IQ) that may drive infant and child outcomes.

How do we get around this issue? Some studies are better than others, and we should look to those for answers. When I looked at the data for the effects of breastfeeding, I tried to tease out the good studies from the less-good ones, and I've based my conclusions only on the better studies. To link most obviously to the example above, a study that is able to adjust for maternal IQ is going to give more believable results than one that isn't.

As you know by now, this book is focused on evidence in the form of data and what we can learn from that data. But there is another type of evidence, one that you see a lot on the internet. I'd refer to this as "things people said" or "it happened once to my friend" evidence. You know: "My friend didn't breastfeed, and her kid went to Harvard." "My friend didn't vaccinate, and her kid is super healthy!"

Here is what we learn from this: nothing.

Heed the statistics mantra: anecdote is not data. (I might put that on a T-shirt.)

Now, as breastfeeding will take us more deeply into questions of data, a word on the types of studies I'll use throughout the book.

AN ASIDE ON
RESEARCH METHODS

When researchers study breastfeeding—or any of the other things I talk about in this book—they are looking to learn about the effect of whatever they are studying while *holding everything else constant.* Our "ideal" experimental setup would be to see a child first after being breastfed, then the same child after not being breastfed, but with everything else exactly the same—same timeline, same parents, same parenting style, same home environment. If we could see that, we would just need to compare the child's later outcomes to know the effects of breastfeeding.

Of course, this is not possible. But when researchers conduct an analysis, this is what they are aiming for. How close they come depends a lot on how good their research methods are.

Randomized Controlled Trial

The "gold standard" for research methods is the randomized controlled trial. To run this kind of study, you recruit some people (ideally a lot of them) and then choose randomly which people will be "treated" as part of your study and which will be the "controls." For a randomized trial of breastfeeding, you'd want to have the "treatment group" breastfeed, and the "control group" not. Since you have chosen randomly who will be in which group, the groups are, on average, the same, other than the breastfeeding. You can then compare what happens for the breastfeeding group with what happens for the control.

A practical challenge with this type of study is that you typically cannot *force* people to do things, especially with their children. Instead, most studies I'll report on use an "encouragement design": One group is encouraged to do the behavior—breastfeed, or sleep train their child, or engage in some discipline program—and the other group is not. This encouragement could, for example, take the form of telling the group about the benefits of that behavior, or giving them some training or guidance about how to accomplish the behavior successfully. Assuming that the encouragement changes how many people do the thing you are studying, you can draw causal conclusions.

Randomized trials are expensive to run, especially if they are big, and they can, of course, have problems with implementation. But they are the closest we're able to come to our ideal treat-the-same-kid-in-two-ways setup, so when I find them, I give them a lot of weight.

Observational Studies

A second, very large group of studies will fall under the "observational study" category. These studies compare, for example, children who are breastfed with those who are not, or those who are sleep trained with those who are not, *without* having randomly assigned people to groups.

The basic structure of these studies is similar. Researchers access (or collect) some data on children, either short- or long-term outcomes, along with some information on parental behaviors. They then analyze the differences between kids in different groups—comparing, say, the kids who are breastfed with the kids who are not.

This type of study will make up the vast majority of the data we have to work with, and they vary widely in quality. One source of variation is study size—some of these are bigger than others, and bigger is typically better. But more important, there will be a lot of variation in how close they can get to the ideal of comparing the same child across one variable in two otherwise identical scenarios.

When they do their comparisons, researchers have to adjust for inherent differences across families that make different parenting choices. Most studies do this by adjusting for some aspects of the parents, or of the child, but their ability to do this well depends on the quality of the data.

On one end, you have sibling studies, which compare two children within the same family who were treated differently on the variable you care about. For example, one of the kids was breastfed, and one was not. Since these children have the same parents and grew up together, there is a strong argument that, other than the breastfeeding, they are similar. These sibling studies are not perfect—you have to ask, why nurse one kid and not the other?—but they have a lot of value in eliminating some of the most important problems in observational studies. There is likely some randomness in the choice to nurse, perhaps related to how much each baby takes to it (I'm thinking of my own experience here).

Many other studies do not compare siblings, but they do see *a lot* of information about parents: education, maybe IQ tests, income, race, other aspects of the home environment, characteristics of the child at birth, etc. Once the authors adjust for these variables, they can get closer to comparing two identical children. I'll often call these variables *controls*. The more things we control for—meaning, the more variables we can hold constant across children and families—the more confident we can be that we are really learning the effects of breastfeeding.

On the other end there are studies that have just one or two controls—that, say, adjust for differences in birth weight across children, but nothing else. These are more suspect.

Case-Control Studies

There is a final class of results that come from what are called case-control studies. These studies tend to be used when there is a rare outcome. Let's say you want to look at the relationship between reading to your child and your child learning to read *very* early (say, before the age of three). Learning to read before three is a very rare outcome. Even in a very large dataset, you might have only a few cases. This isn't enough data to learn about what determines this outcome.

With a case-control approach, researchers start by identifying a set of "cases"—people who had the rare outcome. In our example, that means they go out and actually look for children who could read fluently before age three, and they collect a bunch of data about them. They then look for a set of controls—children who are similar on some dimensions but didn't read until later—and compare them. They ask whether some behavior—in this example, parents reading to the kids—are more common in the children who were early readers.

In general, these studies are worse than the other types. They have, first off, all the same problems as observational studies: the people who are in the case group may be different in many ways from those in the control group, and it is hard to control for those differences. This problem is often more extreme since the control group is typically recruited to the study in a different way from the treatment group.

There are other problems, too. These studies usually rely on asking parents about aspects of their behavior far in the past—parents may struggle to remember, and their memories may be affected by what has happened with their child in the intervening years.

Finally, these studies tend to be small, and the authors are often looking at many possible variables that might be associated with what they are studying. This can lead to spurious conclusions.

There will be times when these are the only studies we have to go on, and we do want to try to learn something from the data they contain. But I tend to approach these with caution.

BACK TO BREASTFEEDING

In the particular case of breastfeeding, we'll see all the kinds of studies described above. There is one large randomized controlled trial of breastfeeding, which was run in Belarus in the 1990s.[6] This study encouraged some women to breastfeed and not others, and there were differences across groups in breastfeeding rates. This study will be relevant for looking at some short-term health outcomes, and some longer-term things like child height and IQ.

There are also some very nice observational studies. There are a few that compare siblings, which is great, and others that were not able to use siblings but do have a large sample size and observe a lot of data about kids and their parents.

Finally, for a few rare and tragic outcomes—childhood cancer, SIDS— we will have to look at some case-control studies, and try to learn what we can from them.

In the rest of this chapter, I'll go through the short- and long-term benefits of breastfeeding to kids and to moms in detail. I will leave aside the issue of methane and say only that it is true that cows produce methane, and it is also true that formula usually contains milk products, so in that sense this benefit is valid.

Oh, and I should say that even if you've decided to breastfeed, making it work is not always easy. To tackle that (stay out of hot closets!), check out the next chapter.

The Benefits

BREASTFEEDING AND EARLY-LIFE HEALTH

Breastfeeding and early-life health is the most well-studied set of relationships. It was the initial focus of the large randomized trial I mentioned earlier, and these are also the relationships with the most compelling set of mechanisms. We know breast milk contains antibodies, so it is therefore more plausible that it is protective against some illnesses.

We'll start with the randomized trial. This study, called PROBIT, was run in Belarus in the 1990s. It followed 17,000 mother-infant pairs across a number of sites in Belarus. The authors started with a sample of women who intended to breastfeed; half of these women were randomly chosen to receive breastfeeding assistance and encouragement. The rest were not discouraged, but they were not provided with support.

The encouragement had a big effect on breastfeeding. At three months, 43 percent of children of moms who were encouraged were exclusively breastfed, versus just 6 percent of children whose mothers were not. There were also differences in whether the babies got any breast milk at this point. At a year, the any-breastfeeding rates were 20 percent and 11 percent, suggesting that the effects of the encouragement persisted.[7]

You'll notice that the encouragement didn't mean *all* the moms who were encouraged to breastfeed did, or that all the moms who were not encouraged didn't. The results, then, may be smaller than they would be if there were a larger difference in breastfeeding between the two groups.[8]

The study found two significant impacts: In the first year, breastfed babies had fewer gastrointestinal infections (i.e., diarrhea) and lower rates of eczema and other rashes. To put some numbers to it, 13 percent of the children of mothers in the group that wasn't encouraged to breastfeed had at least one diarrhea episode, versus only 9 percent of those whose mothers were encouraged. The rate of rashes and eczema was also lower in the group whose mothers were encouraged to breastfeed: 3 percent versus 6 percent.

These effects are significant, and as a share of the overall rates of these illnesses, they are reasonably big. For example, rashes and eczema were reduced by half. Having said that, the overall rates are worth keeping in perspective: even in the group that breastfed less, only 6 percent of children were reported to have this complication. It is also important to note that these are typically fairly minor illnesses.

There is one very serious early-life illness—also linked to digestion—that seems to be affected by breast milk. Necrotizing enterocolitis (NEC) is a serious intestinal complication that is a risk for very preterm babies (it is most common for babies weighing less than three and a half pounds at birth). Breast milk (from either the mother or a donor) has been shown to lower the risk of this condition in randomized trials.[9] This may bolster our confidence in the general links with digestion, although for full-term (or even nearly full-term) babies, NEC is vanishingly rare.

In the PROBIT trial, there were also many illness measures that didn't seem to be affected by breastfeeding, including respiratory infections, ear infections, croup, and wheezing. Indeed, the share of kids in each group who had these problems was virtually identical. It is important to be clear on what this means. It does not mean we are *sure* breastfeeding has absolutely no effect on respiratory problems. These estimates come with statistical errors, what we call "confidence intervals," which give us a sense of how sure we are about the estimate we observe. In this particular study, we cannot reject the possibility that breastfeeding could matter in either direction—that it could decrease or increase respiratory infections.

What we *can* say is that the data doesn't support the claim of a reduction in respiratory infections as a result of breastfeeding.

Given these findings, why do we continue to see the "evidence-based" claim that breastfeeding reduces colds and ear infections? The main reason is there are many observational studies—which compare kids who are breastfed with those who are not, but not where breastfeeding is randomly varied—that do show that breastfeeding affects these illnesses. An especially large set of studies argues for an effect of breastfeeding on ear infections.[10]

Should we give any weight to this evidence once we have a randomized trial?

This is a complicated question. On one hand, all things being equal, randomized evidence is clearly better. We know that breastfeeding is not something people do on a whim, and we know that women who nurse have different circumstances from those who do not. This leads us to favor the randomized evidence.

On the other hand, the randomized trial is only one study. And it is not infinitely large. If there are small benefits from breastfeeding, they might not show up as significant effects in the randomized trial, but we would still like to know about them. I think it is reasonable, therefore, to look at the non-randomized data, especially when it comes to ear infections, which are widely studied, and where some of the evidence comes from very large and high-quality datasets.

For example, a study of 70,000 Danish women published in 2016 found that breastfeeding through six months reduced the risk of an ear infection from 7 percent to 5 percent over those months.[11] This study was very careful and complete, with excellent data that allowed the authors to adjust for a lot of differences across mothers and children.

This effect isn't replicated everywhere. A similar study in the UK shows no impact on ear infections.[12] But in my view, the weight of overall evidence puts this in the plausible category.

In contrast, there isn't any study as compelling as this Danish ear infection study on colds and coughs. The studies on these symptoms are smaller and less statistically convincing, and the results are fragile. There seems to be less to learn here.

Where does this leave us? Certainly, it seems reasonable to conclude that breastfeeding lowers infant eczema and gastrointestinal infections. For the other illness outcomes, the most compelling evidence is in favor of a small reduction in ear infections in breastfed children.

BREASTFEEDING AND SIDS

I would be remiss to leave the discussion of breast milk and early-life health without discussing the relationship between breastfeeding and SIDS, the tragic cases in which an infant dies unexpectedly in the crib. The relationship of SIDS to breastfeeding, while frequently posited, is difficult to untangle.

The death of a child is among the worst things you can imagine as a parent. In this book, we will look at many questions that feel weighted, but nothing will compare to this horrific circumstance. This gives added emotional valence to even the suggested possibility of a relationship between breastfeeding and infant mortality.

SIDS is rare; ear infections and colds are common. Your kids will get colds for sure, whether you breastfeed or not. SIDS deaths, in contrast, occur in about 1 of every 1,800 births; among babies with no other risk factors (not premature, not sleeping on their stomachs), this is perhaps 1 in 10,000.[13]

This should reassure anxious parents to some extent, but it also makes the SIDS–breastfeeding relationship hard to study, since you need an enormously large sample of babies to learn anything that can benefit other children.

To get around this, studies of this relationship use the case-control method: They identify a number of infants who have died of SIDS, interview the parents, then interview a set of control parents with living children. The characteristics of the parents and children are compared.

There are many of these studies.[14] And, on average, they do find that the living children are more likely to be breastfed. This causes them to conclude that not breastfeeding increases the risk of SIDS. The most recent analyses suggest that these effects are most pronounced for breastfeeding longer than two months.[15]

In my opinion, however, from a careful read of the data, this conclusion is not obvious. There are basic differences between the children who die and those who do not, differences that likely have nothing to do with breastfeeding but are driving many of the results. When the studies take into account things like a parent's smoking, whether the baby was premature, and other risk factors—all of which are correlated with breastfeeding and linked to SIDS—their effects are much smaller or disappear altogether.

Beyond this, some of the research papers with the largest effects also have a serious problem with their selection of the control group. A key component of designing these studies is to pick a control group that is as comparable as possible, and these studies are not always successful in this goal.

For example, it is common to select all infants who die of SIDS in an area as the treatment group, and then recruit parents of living children with letters or phone calls. But this means the people in the control group are chosen differently, and we know that people who want to participate in a study are fundamentally different—in ways we can see and ways we cannot—from people who do not choose to be involved.[16]

Reinforcing this concern, studies with a better selection of control babies—for example, one where the comparison group comprises babies who were visited by the same home-visiting nurse in England—do not show an elevated risk of SIDS from not breastfeeding.[17]

SIDS deaths are thankfully rare. Because they are so rare, it is impossible to fully rule out the possibility that breastfeeding decreases the risk of SIDS by a small amount. However, I do not believe the best data supports a significant link.

BREASTFEEDING AND LATER HEALTH

Most of the academic research on breastfeeding focuses on early-life outcomes—infections, for example, in the time period in which you might actually be breastfeeding. In the popular discourse, however, the focus seems to be much more on the long-term benefits. This is where the guilt stacks up.

You rarely hear people say, "It's great to breastfeed since it lowers the chances of diarrhea in the next six months!" Rather, they say things like, "It's great to breastfeed since that gives your kid the best start; they'll be smarter, taller, thinner!" This problem isn't limited to random people on the street: one woman told me her doctor had told her that by quitting breastfeeding, she was costing her child three IQ points.

The idea that choosing not to breastfeed might be something your child would suffer from for their whole life is far worse as a parent than simply thinking they might get one more ear infection.

The good news for guilt-ridden moms is that, even more than in the case of early-life health issues, I have not seen any convincing evidence for these long-term impacts.

We can begin with the set of outcomes studied in PROBIT. These researchers have continued to follow the children in the trial through the age of seven. They find no evidence of any long-term health impacts: no change in allergies or asthma, cavities, height, blood pressure, weight, or indicators for being overweight or obese.[18]

The results on obesity are worth pausing on, as this benefit of breastfeeding gets a lot of attention. (When I was pregnant with Finn, there was a very large poster in my midwife's office claiming that breastfeeding lowered obesity, a message underscored by the image of two ice cream scoops, each topped with a cherry so they looked like breasts. It was a neat visual, although the point it was illustrating remains unclear to me. I suppose the idea was that you could eat more ice cream if you were breastfed.)

It is certainly true that obesity and breastfeeding are correlated, as kids who are breastfed are less likely to be obese later in life. But this correlation doesn't show causation—it doesn't prove that those kids who go on to become obese do so *because* they weren't breastfed. The randomized data from PROBIT shows no impact of breastfeeding on whether the child is obese at the age of seven or, in the latest follow-up, at close to eleven.[19] Bolstering this, studies that compare siblings who are breastfed to those who are not show no differences in obesity. These studies often demonstrate that breastfeeding seems to matter when you compare across families, but not *within* a family. This suggests that something about the family, not the breastfeeding, is impacting the likelihood of a child becoming obese.[20] In fact, when researchers look at many studies of obesity and breastfeeding together to get a fuller picture, they find that studies that carefully adjust for maternal socioeconomic status, maternal smoking, and maternal weight—even if they cannot compare siblings—also show no association.[21]

All these results come with some statistical error. Can we say *for sure* that breastfeeding does not impact obesity? No. But we can say that nothing compelling in the data supports a significant link.

A few long-term outcomes—for example, juvenile arthritis and urinary tract infections—could not be studied in PROBIT, but at least one or two studies have shown some link between these conditions and breastfeeding. The evidence on most of these links is simply very limited.[22] A significant relationship shows up in only one of many studies, or the research design is poor, or the population is very unusual—basically, we cannot learn anything from the data about whether there is a relationship.

More has been written on two more serious illnesses—type 1 diabetes and childhood cancer—but, again, given the limitations of the data, I do not think we learn much. More on these two in the endnote.[23]

In many of these cases—like others in the breastfeeding arena—even very limited and poorly done studies get a lot of attention. Media attention tends to miss the nuance of published literature, even when the literature itself is good, which is often not the case. We see, again and again, aggressive headlines that often overstate the claims of the articles they report on.

Why is this?

One reason is that people seem to love a scary or shocking narrative. "Report: Formula-Fed Children More Likely to Drop Out of High School" is a more clickable headline than "Large, Well-Designed Study Shows Small Impacts of Breastfeeding on Diarrheal Diseases." This desire for shock and awe interacts poorly with most people's lack of statistical knowledge. There is no pressure on the media to focus on reporting the "best" studies, since people have a hard time separating the good studies from the less-good ones. Media reports can get away with saying "A new study shows . . ." without saying "A new study, with very likely biased results, shows..." And other than the few of us who get our dander up on Twitter, people are mostly none the wiser.

It is hard to sort out study quality from this initial media coverage, although it's probably easier in the age of the internet. Many media reports will now link to the original study. If the "Formula-Fed Children More Likely to Drop Out of High School" article is based on a study of forty-five people surveyed about their breastfeeding behavior when their now twenty-year-old children were infants, you can probably let it go.

SMARTY-BOOBS: BREASTFEEDING AND IQ

Breast milk is optimal for brain development, right? Nurse your way to a successful child! So they say. But is this true? Will breast milk make your kid smarter?

Let's start by returning from the land of magical breast milk to reality. Even in the most optimistic view about breastfeeding, the impact on IQ is small. Breastfeeding isn't going to increase your child's IQ by twenty points. How do we know? Because if it did, it would be really obvious in the data and in your everyday experience.

The question is, really, whether breastfeeding gives children some small leg up in intelligence. If you believe studies that just compare kids who are breastfed to those who are not, you find that it does. I talked about one example of these studies on page 68, and there are others. There is a clear correlation here—breastfed kids do seem to have higher IQs.

But this isn't the same as saying that breastfeeding *causes* the higher IQ. In reality, the causal link is much more tenuous. We can see this by looking carefully at a number of studies that compare children who were breastfed to their siblings who were not. These studies tend to find no relationship between breastfeeding and IQ. The children who were nursed did no better on IQ tests than their siblings who were not.

This conclusion differs fundamentally from the studies without sibling comparisons. One very nice study gives us an answer to why.[24] The key to this study is that the authors analyze the same sample of kids in a bunch of different ways. First, they compare children who are breastfed with those who are not with a few simple controls. When they do this, they find large differences in child IQ between the breastfed kids and those who are not. In the second phase, they add an adjustment for the mother's IQ, and find that the effect of breastfeeding is much smaller—much of the effect attributed to breastfeeding in the first analysis was due to differences in the mothers' IQs—but does still persist.

But then the authors do a third analysis where they compare siblings—children born to the same mother—one of whom was breastfed and one who was not. This is valuable because it takes into account *all* the differences between the moms, not just their performance on one IQ test. In this analysis, researchers see that breastfeeding doesn't have a significant impact on IQ. This suggests that it is something about the mother (or the parents in general), not anything about breast milk, that is driving the breastfeeding effect in the first analysis.

PROBIT also looked at the relationship between breastfeeding and IQ. For this sample, the measurement of IQ was done by researchers who knew whether a child was in the breastfeeding-encouraged treatment group. There were no significant effects of breastfeeding on overall IQ or on teachers' evaluations of the children's performance in school. The researchers did see small impacts of breastfeeding on verbal IQ in some of their tests, but further analysis suggested that this may have been driven by the people doing the measurement—knowing which children were breastfed might have influenced their evaluation.[25] Overall, therefore, this study doesn't provide especially strong support for the claim that breast-feeding increases IQ.[26]

In conclusion, there is no compelling evidence for smarty-boobs.

BENEFITS FOR MOM

For some women, breastfeeding makes them feel empowered and happy. It's convenient to have a ready food source anywhere they go, and they find nursing their baby to be a peaceful and relaxing time. That's great!

For others, breastfeeding makes them feel like a cow. They hate lugging the breast pump around if they have to pump. It's hard to tell if the baby even likes to nurse or is getting enough food. Their nipples hurt, and the experience basically sucks.

All this is to say that many of the purported benefits of breastfeeding for moms are really subjective. I have been on both sides of this, as have most of my friends. There were definitely moments—especially with Finn—when I thought it was a superconvenient and awesome option. And then there were others—I am thinking in particular of an experience pumping in the bathroom at LaGuardia Airport—when the whole thing seemed like a farce.

One of the things on every pro-breastfeeding list is "saves money." This really depends. Yes, formula is expensive, but so are nursing tops, nipple creams, nursing pads, and the fourteen different breastfeeding pillows you need to make it work. And, more important, there is your time, which is valuable.

Another claimed benefit is "stress resistance." Does breastfeeding make you more resistant to stress? Again, pretty subjective. Stress is very often linked with sleep disturbance. Will you get more sleep if you nurse your baby? This depends on more than just breastfeeding.

As mentioned earlier, "better friendships" has also been touted as a benefit. You'll need to decide for yourself if your friendships will be enhanced by breastfeeding. (It probably depends on your friends.)

These are just a few of the "benefits" of breastfeeding for which there is just no evidence. A few claimed benefits, however, do potentially have some basis in fact. The first is the claim that breastfeeding is "free birth control." Here is the truth: you are less likely to get pregnant if you breastfeed, but it is not—I repeat, *NOT*—a reliable birth control method, especially as your child ages and if you ever go more than a few hours without feeding or pumping. I do not have enough space in this book to list all the people I know who got pregnant while breastfeeding (shout-out here to my medical editor, Adam, his wife, and his second child). If you definitely do not want to get pregnant, you need to use some real birth control.

A second claimed benefit with some evidence is "weight loss." I'm sorry to report that, at best, any weight loss effects are small. One large study from North Carolina showed that at three months postpartum, weight loss was similar in moms who breastfed and those who did not. At six months postpartum, the breastfeeding moms had lost about 1.4 pounds more.[27] Issues with this paper mean this is likely an overestimate of the effect of breastfeeding on weight loss, but at any rate, it is still very small.

You may be wondering, *Doesn't breastfeeding burn calories? Didn't I hear something about how you use five hundred calories a day nursing?* This is true, but women who are nursing tend to eat more. Burning more calories is effective as a weight-loss strategy only if you do not make those calories up in what you eat. When I was nursing, I had a policy of eating an egg and cheese bagel sandwich at ten thirty every morning. This type of behavior pretty much guarantees you will replace the calories you burn.

The evidence of the effect of breastfeeding on postpartum depression is similarly noncompelling. Studies of this relationship show mixed results, and it's a hard question to evaluate since the causality goes both ways. Mothers suffering from postpartum depression are more likely to quit breastfeeding, which makes it look like breastfeeding relieves postpartum depression, when actually, the causality is the other way around.[28] And the claim of lowered risk of developing osteoporosis and improved bone health is also not apparent in large datasets.[29] Evidence on diabetes is also mixed, and likely confounded with differences across women.

There is one benefit that does have a larger and more robust evidence base: the link between breastfeeding and cancers, in particular breast cancer. Across a wide variety of studies and locations, there seems to be a relationship here, and a sizable one—perhaps a 20 to 30 percent reduction in the risk of breast cancer. Breast cancer is a common cancer—almost 1 in 8 women will have a form of it at some point in their lives—so this reduction is big in absolute terms.

This data isn't perfect—for one thing, the controls for maternal socioeconomic status are almost always missing—but the case for causality is bolstered by a concrete set of mechanisms. Breastfeeding changes some aspects of the cells of the breast, which makes them less susceptible to carcinogens. In addition, breastfeeding lowers estrogen production, which in turn can lower the risk of breast cancer.

After all that focus on the benefits of breastfeeding for kids, it may be that the most important long-term impact is actually on *Mom's* health.

THE VERDICT

We can now return, at long last, to our table of significant benefits, and try to weed out those for which we did not find compelling evidence.

In some cases, things drop out of the table because there is simply no data on them—better friendships, for example. It's not that we have compelling evidence to reject this, it's just that no one has actually run any studies about it. In other cases—obesity, say—the facts show that people have studied this, and the best data doesn't support a link.

For the relationships that were dropped from the table, nothing in the data suggests they are really linked. Put differently, you might equally plausibly link breastfeeding to a wide variety of other outcomes—being a fast runner or good at playing the violin. This doesn't mean it can't be true, just that there is nothing in the data to suggest it is. You can take the relationship on faith, but you shouldn't take it as evidence.

Our list of benefits supported by evidence is now more limited,

Short-Term Baby Benefits	Long-Term Child Benefits: Health	Long-Term Child Benefits: Cognitive	Benefits for Mom	Benefits for World
▪ Fewer allergic rashes ▪ Fewer gastro-intestinal disorders ▪ Lower risk of NEC ▪ Fewer ear infections (maybe)			▪ Lower risk of breast cancer	▪ Lower methane produc-tion from cows

although not entirely empty. There do seem to be some short-term bene-fits for your baby, and maybe some longer-term benefits for you. And don't forget the methane! But relative to the initial list, this one is a lot shorter.

The pressure on moms to breastfeed can be immense. The rhetoric makes it seem like this is the most important thing you can—and need—to do to set your child up for success. Breastfeeding is magic! Milk is liquid gold!

This just isn't right. Yes, if you want to breastfeed, great! But while there are some short-term benefits for your baby, if you don't want to nurse, or if it doesn't work out, it's not a tragedy for your baby, or for you. It is almost certainly worse if you spend a year sitting around feeling bad about not nursing.

When I was writing this book, I looked back at the books my mother and grandmother used when they had children. My mother was a fan of *Dr. Spock's Baby and Child Care*, a book written in the 1940s and updated periodically; I have her version from the mid-1980s.

Dr. Spock addresses the issue of breastfeeding by suggesting that moms try it to see if they like it. He says something brief about possible protection from infection for babies, and then says, "The most convincing evidence on the value of breastfeeding comes from mothers who have done it. They tell of the tremendous satisfaction they experience from knowing that they are providing their babies with something no one else can give them . . . from feeling their closeness."

At least for me, this resonated very strongly. I am happy I nursed my children because—aside from some of the early hot-closet incidents—I enjoyed it. It made for many nice moments with them, doing something we could only do together, watching them fall asleep. This is a great reason to do it, and a good reason to try. It's also a good reason to support women who want to try, and to not shame women who breastfeed in public. But this is not a good reason to judge yourself if you decide breastfeeding isn't for you.

The Bottom Line

- There are some health benefits to breastfeeding early on, although the evidence supporting them is more limited than is commonly stated.
- There are likely some long-term health benefits, related to breast cancer, for Mom.
- The data does not provide strong evidence for long-term health or cognitive benefits of breastfeeding for your child.

Breastfeeding:
A How-To Guide

When I think back on my first weeks of breastfeeding Penelope, they are mostly a haze of frustration.

At the time, I felt like I had all the breastfeeding problems. The latching problem. The supply problem. I would nurse and nurse and then every night we'd have to feed Penelope a huge bottle, which she sucked down, seemingly judging me for not having enough milk (I might have been imagining that). Then there was the pump: When to pump? How often, early on? Once I was back at work, how was I supposed to relax enough to pump? Can you pump on a conference call? Only if you mute it?

It can feel like you are the only person with these problems. This is especially true at the beginning, when it's hard to make breastfeeding work. The hours of sitting alone in a room with a newborn, trying to get them to eat—it's isolating. This is exacerbated by the fact that all the breastfeeding moms you see—the ones walking around the farmers' market nursing their infants—seem to be having no problem carrying a bag of corn, herding their three-year-old past the cookie display, and feeding their baby. Maybe you *are* the only one with problems.

You are not. In writing this chapter, I appealed to Twitter: Fellow moms, tell me your breastfeeding woes.

They had a lot to say.

People told me about trying and trying to get their babies to latch, without success. They told me about their "stupid tiny nipples" and the time they bought a "booby tube" (Google it). About painful nipples—bleeding, cracked, and, in one especially gory case, actually partially coming off.

People told me about supply issues. Undersupply—the time one woman sent her husband on a thirty-minute bus ride to get her nettle tea *right now*, or the constant attempts to increase supply by nursing and then pumping twelve times a day, after every feeding. Oversupply—leaky breasts getting milk on everything; mattresses smelling of Parmesan and clothes stiff with dried milk. One woman told me she had an undersupply of milk, yet started spurting milk on the bus every time a baby cried.

And then there was the pump. "Pumping is the worst" filled my email inbox. One woman said she lost her fingerprints from transferring sterilized pump parts to a drying rack. People wrote of feeling isolated and falling behind at their jobs because of the hours they spent shut in their offices pumping, of the embarrassment of asking for pumping time on business trips, or pumping in the bathroom since there was no other place to do it. And they told of the frustration of not getting enough milk, even with all their effort.

I can perhaps be accused of armchair psychology here, but these struggles seem particularly acute because trying harder—something that usually breeds success—doesn't always work with breastfeeding. You worked hard to get a job, or to get into college—even to get pregnant—and you were successful! But introduce a new person, and some further constraints of biology, and all bets are off. You may have to accept, as I did, that no matter how hard you try, you will not make quite enough milk.

It is not helpful that this is a surprise for many women, who thought, *Hey, billions of people do this, how hard can it be?* When I asked, many women expressed the wish that they had known it could be *so* hard and had not felt such shame and pressure to continue. For that, I refer you to the previous chapter. Here, let's leave it at this: Breastfeeding is hard for many women, and many women struggle with it, especially with their first child. If you are one of them, you are not alone. There is some evidence that might help in the pages that follow—and giving yourself a break will help, too.

GENERAL INTERVENTIONS

If, like many breastfeeding women, you have faced these challenges, you have likely heard about many different strategies to overcome them. Some of these strategies seem reasonable, some not so much. What does the data say?

Evidence on causes of breastfeeding success can really be divided into two categories. There are some specific questions: Do nipple shields work? Will fenugreek increase your milk supply? And there are more general questions: Is there anything you can plan on before birth that might increase your likelihood of breastfeeding success?

The broad answer to this second question is yes, there are two evidence-supported things you can do. We'll start with these.

First, there is some randomized evidence on the success of skin-to-skin contact at improving breastfeeding success rates. Skin-to-skin contact is the practice of having women hold their naked (or diapered) baby against their naked chest, typically right after birth. The idea is that the smells and the proximity will encourage the baby to start feeding immediately. Much of this evidence comes from developing countries, where the overall breastfeeding rates are different and technologies around birth may also be different. Nevertheless, breastfeeding is a universal human experience, so there is no reason we cannot learn from the experiences of women in these countries. One study of two hundred women in India randomized the mothers into either holding their infant skin to skin for forty-five minutes after birth or having them in an infant warmer.[1] The moms who had their infants skin to skin were more likely (72 percent versus 57 percent) to be breastfeeding at six weeks; they also reported less pain while being stitched up after birth.

These results are confirmed by a review of a large number of small studies.[2] Putting them together, breastfeeding initiation and success seem to be higher with skin-to-skin contact, including after a caesarean section.

Second, there is some (more limited) evidence that breastfeeding support—by a doctor, or by a nurse or lactation consultant—can increase likelihood of breastfeeding initiation and continuation.[3] This evidence comes from a wide variety of studies of different types of interventions. Because not all the interventions are the same, it is hard to pinpoint precisely what is useful. The basic principle is that it can take time to learn to nurse, and having assistance from someone who has seen it before may help you work past some of the obvious problems. It may simply be helpful to have someone to strategize with, ideally someone who has slept in the past few days and can provide some perspective. (This can, by the way, help with a lot of decisions about your newborn.)

A couple of small studies focus on hospital versus in-home education, and find some additional benefits from getting help once you're home from the hospital.[4] The hospital environment is not your own, and having someone come to your home to help you figure out what you are doing can be hugely useful.

Anecdotally, breastfeeding support at the hospital can be hit or miss. Some women described their lactation consultants as judgmental and mean. Others thought they were great. If you are not getting the help you need, keep asking to see if you can find the right person. If you can manage it, getting this help from someone you know and trust—a doula, or perhaps a lactation consultant you've talked to before the birth about what you want—may be the most helpful.

A final general intervention that deserves mention is rooming in at the hospital. As discussed in an earlier chapter (see page 15), there is no evidence that this enhances the likelihood of breastfeeding success.[5]

LATCHING ON

If you are planning to breastfeed, the first challenge is the latch. In order to efficiently get milk from the breast, your baby needs to open their mouth pretty wide and get your whole nipple in their mouth; they then use their tongue and lips to suck. Contrary to what I had envisioned, it is not like they are delicately sipping the end of the nipple. In the words of my friend Jane, "You really have to jam the kid on there."

There is a picture below that captures the fact that the baby needs to get a whole mouthful of boob, although not that you have to jam them on. I will say that until you see it for yourself with an actual baby, it's tough to visualize.

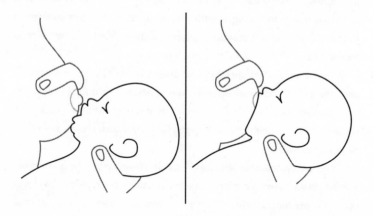

Many infants struggle to latch on correctly. Without a good latch, the baby will not get enough milk, and it can be extremely painful for Mom. How do you know you have a good latch? Once you have done it for a while, you'll just know. You'll also learn to recognize a kind of weird sigh that many babies have when they get it right. Before that . . . it is useful to have someone else look and tell you. The internet will tell you that if you have a good latch, nursing will not hurt. More on this later, but for now, know that early on, this is often not true. For many women, breastfeeding will hurt for the first couple of weeks whether the baby is latched well or not, so you cannot reliably use pain as a signal.

Why might infants have trouble latching? Prematurity, illness, or birth injury could be the cause. It could also have to do with their mother's nipples—some women have inverted nipples that can make latching difficult. Finally, some infants have structural issues in their mouths—in particular, conditions called tongue tie or lip tie—that make it difficult to latch.

Or maybe your baby hates you! Ha, I'm kidding. It will only feel like that.

One solution to this problem—at least to some extent—is to keep trying with someone around to help you. Here is where a doula or other support person might come in. Most people do get the hang of this, but being patient with yourself is likely to make it go better.

If you have prolonged problems with latching, there are two common interventions: nipple shields and a (quick) surgical procedure to address tongue tie.

Many women swear by nipple shields, at least early on. The name is pretty descriptive: they are shaped like a nipple, typically made of silicone, with little holes in them. You put the shield over the nipple, and the infant sucks on that. These shields can make it easier for infants to latch, in principle, and make nursing less painful for Mom.

The main downside of the nipple shield, other than that it is annoying to wash, is that it affects milk transfer. The shield reduces stimulation, so your body produces less milk.[6] There is a clear physiological basis for this, and it has been shown in randomized trials.

This doesn't answer the question of whether nipple shields are effective, though, since the point isn't to increase milk transfer but to get the baby on the breast in the first place. Unfortunately, there is no very good evidence on whether they work. The best study we have is of thirty-four premature infants, in which researchers had access to information on how much milk they got with and without the shield. This study found that infants got way more milk with the shield than without—more than four times as much—which is encouraging. But, again, this study wasn't randomized, the sample was tiny, and it focused on a particular population.[7]

What we do have as evidence is a lot of qualitative work in which women are interviewed about their experiences with using nipple shields, and they do credit the shields with allowing them to continue breastfeeding and working through issues like pain and latching problems.[8] There is an implicit counterfactual here—that they would have quit without the shield—although it is hard to know if this is right.

The downside of trying nipple shields is that it can be difficult to quit using them—if you and your baby get used to them, it might be hard to transition off. This is okay if you are happy using them and your baby is getting enough milk, but it does add another step to the feeding process. So it is probably not a first-line defense—as in, not everyone should start with these. On the other hand, if things are not working, they're a good option to try.

A more involved intervention is a surgical procedure to address tongue tie or lip tie in infants. This suggestion will come up only if your infant actually has a tongue or lip tie. The tongue attaches to the floor of the mouth with a cord called the frenulum. In some people, this cord is very short, which can limit tongue mobility. For infants, this can affect the ability to breastfeed, since the mechanics rely on the tongue. Tongue tie is thought to be reasonably common, and in serious cases can affect speech later in a child's life. Lip tie refers to a similar (but less common) condition in which the cord that attaches the upper lip to the gums is short, or placed very low, limiting lip mobility.

There is a simple surgical solution to either condition, which is to snip the cord, releasing the tongue or lip and allowing it to move more freely. The surgery is common and safe, and mechanically it does seem like it could be effective.[9]

The evidence in favor of realized success, though, is fairly limited. There are four randomized trials of this procedure, all of them very small, and only three of which evaluate its impact on feeding success.[10] Among these, two showed no difference in feeding success, and one showed improvements. All four studies did show improvements in maternal pain during nursing, although this was self-reported. The limited evidence suggests that this procedure, even more so than nipple shields, shouldn't be a first-line defense, even in cases where some tongue tie is present.

For most women, even those whose babies latch well, breastfeeding is at least somewhat painful early on. Any pain should be mostly gone after the first minute or two of nursing, not continue. Certain conditions can cause ongoing pain—for example, nipple yeast infections—but are treatable. It would be a shame not to figure that out, so if your pain persists, ask for help.

Nipples can become cracked and sore, or bleed. There is no magic solution to fix this problem. Many women swear by lanolin cream or various gel packs and pads, but there is no randomized evidence suggesting that any of these things are successful.[11] The only thing with any support in randomized trials is the practice of rubbing breast milk on your nipples regularly. I will caution, however, that this data comes from just one trial, and it is small.[12]

Of course, there is no reason not to use lanolin or to rub breast milk on your nipples, so if you feel like that works, or you want to try it, awesome. My friend Hilary, when I asked her about this, wrote me: "MOISTURIZE THE NIPS EVERY TIME."

The very good news is that for most women, regardless of what actions they take, nipple pain does resolve, or at least lessen to manageable levels, after a couple of weeks. This is based on evidence from trials where women had reasonably severe nipple trauma—bleeding, open sores—so even if things look very grim, remember that in most cases, they will resolve themselves.[13]

This evidence also says that still having agonizing pain after two weeks is not typical, nor is it something that should be dismissed with "Oh, it will get better if you keep trying." If you're experiencing this, get help. Many states have breastfeeding hotlines, and La Leche League can often connect you with a lactation specialist over the phone if you do not want to go as far as seeing someone in person.

Nipple pain is different from mastitis, an infection you can get at any time during nursing. Some things will increase the risk of mastitis—including not fully emptying the breasts with each feeding, having an oversupply, or not emptying the breasts frequently enough—but its onset is largely random. It is not hard to diagnose—the symptoms are a red, painful, swollen breast and a high fever—and may need to be treated with antibiotics. Mastitis can be extremely painful and is not something to ignore.

NIPPLE CONFUSION

If you are considering breastfeeding, you will have heard about the dreaded nipple confusion. Many sources will tell you to be very careful about using artificial nipples—on a bottle or a pacifier—since babies will become confused and decide not to latch on to the breast.

In this discussion, it seems important to separate bottle-feeding—where the baby is learning that food can come from another source—and pacifiers, which do not produce food.

Despite the warnings, there is simply no evidence that the use of pacifiers impacts breastfeeding success. This has been shown by more than one randomized trial,[14] including trials that start infants on a pacifier at birth. At least one of these trials gives a sense of why someone might have (incorrectly) concluded that pacifier use matters for breastfeeding. This trial enrolled 281 women and counseled them either in favor of or against pacifier use. Pacifier use was less in the group that was discouraged from it.[15] The main analysis in the paper—which is shown in the first two bars of the graph on page 97—compared breastfeeding rates at three months for women in the pacifier encouragement group with the pacifier discouragement group. This analysis showed no impact of the intervention on breastfeeding rates. In both groups, about 80 percent of moms were nursing at three months, even though one group was much more likely to also use a pacifier with their babies.

The authors then do something clever, which is to compare breastfeeding rates at three months for moms who chose to use a pacifier versus not, *without* using the randomization. Basically, they treat the data as if they didn't have a randomized trial at all, and just saw breastfeeding and pacifier-use rates for mothers.

The results from this analysis are in the second set of bars in the graph below. Here we see that moms who use a pacifier are less likely to be breastfeeding at three months. The researchers' conclusion—comparing the two sets of results—is that some other factor causes both the pacifier use and the early cessation of breastfeeding. For example, given the rhetoric around pacifiers, it is easy to believe that women who choose to use pacifiers may have a less intense desire to breastfeed.

We should base our conclusions on the randomized data, which tells us that pacifier use doesn't affect breastfeeding success. But since much of the rest of the evidence in the literature is based on these observational

CHANCE OF BREASTFEEDING AT 3 MONTHS BY PACIFIER USE

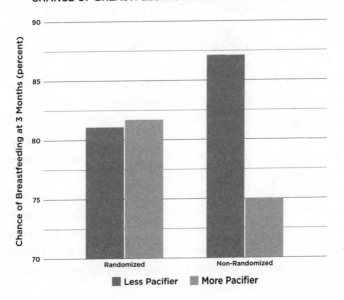

correlations, it is not surprising that people have bought into the myth of pacifiers causing nipple confusion.

Evaluating the role of bottle-feeding nipple confusion is more complicated because there are two factors: the role of supplementing with formula, and the role of nipple confusion. Imagine that breastfeeding success is associated with supplementation—say, because women who have a harder time nursing are more likely to supplement. You will then find that infants who are fed by a bottle early on are less likely to be breastfed in the long run, but this could have nothing to do with the nipple.

A very nice randomized trial addresses this issue using a simple design.[16] Infants needing supplementation are randomized into either supplementation with a bottle or supplementation with a cup, where nipple confusion is not thought to be an issue.[17] These authors found that overall, the method of supplementation did not matter. Both groups had breastfeeding durations of around four months, and exclusive breastfeeding for two to three weeks. Bottle or cup, the results were the same, suggesting that nipple confusion was not an issue.

MILK SUPPLY

My mother had her trusty Dr. Spock book in the 1980s. My *mormor* (grandmother) had her own guide: a set of six little books called *The Mother's Encyclopedia*, first published in 1933. The book makes for great reading. It covers everything from measles to appendicitis to summer camp. Even better, it's in alphabetical order, so you get a discussion of caesarean section followed immediately by a section on competitive sports.

The discussion of breastfeeding in this book spends a large amount of time on the question of supply and, in particular, notes that many "modern" women have trouble producing enough milk. The book blames the recommendation that women nurse only every four hours, and only from one breast. Perhaps the best part is the discussion of "primitive" mothers (their words, not mine) who "nurse their babies when they cry—on any and all occasions!"

The authors note that this "primitive" method is very good for milk supply, although they caution that no one would ever recommend that modern parents return to this approach. It's a good lesson in how things change; generally, the recommendation now is to nurse on demand, at least early on, since this establishes a plentiful milk supply. Schedules, to the extent we get them, come later.

A biological mechanism links the frequency of feeding to milk supply. The system is designed to have a feedback loop where you produce more milk when the baby needs more. The existence of this loop is why, for example, people who are looking to increase their supply will sometimes pump after feedings to trick the body into thinking demand is greater than it is.

Despite a basically reasonable evolutionary design, this doesn't always work quite as planned. First, it can take a lot of time for your milk to start flowing. Second, even once there is milk, you can have an undersupply. And third, on the opposite end, you can have an oversupply.

When your baby is first born, you'll produce a small amount of colostrum, an antibody-rich substance. (You'll actually start producing this in late pregnancy.) Over the first few days, as you nurse, your body will eventually (in theory) switch over from producing colostrum to producing milk in more copious amounts. The expectation is that this switch to more full milk production—scientifically termed lactogenesis II, and sometimes referred to as your milk "coming in"—will occur within the first seventy-two hours after you've given birth. If this doesn't happen, you will be deemed as having "delayed lactogenesis."

In fact, it does take longer than that for many women. The graph on page 100—from a study of 2,500 women—shows the distribution of days from baby's birth to milk production. Almost a quarter of women have milk production delayed beyond three days. This is even higher—about 35 percent—for first-time mothers.[18]

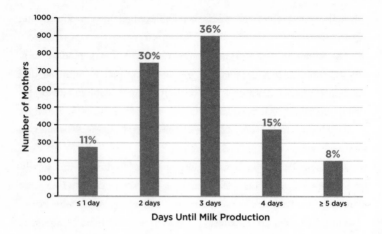

Delayed onset of milk does—in the data—correlate with a higher likelihood of earlier breastfeeding cessation.[19] This may be because delayed onset of milk leads to excess infant weight loss, which makes it harder to get breastfeeding going. It may also be that if you are not especially committed to breastfeeding in the first place, this setback is enough to turn you off from it altogether.

Regardless of whether it is causal, delayed milk onset can be extremely frustrating. There are a few factors that correlate with it.[20]

Smoking during pregnancy slows down milk production, as does obesity. Women who have a caesarean section are more likely to have later onset, as are those who have an epidural during labor. In terms of postbirth modifiable behaviors, both feeding on demand and initiating breastfeeding within an hour of birth are associated with a lower likelihood of delayed milk onset. It is worth emphasizing that these are correlations, not necessarily causal links, and for something like the epidural there may be good reasons to do it anyway. And even if you do everything as suggested, your milk may still be delayed.

Once the milk has arrived, there still may not be enough of it—or there may be too much.

For women who do not have enough supply, a first-line suggestion is

generally to try to use the "demand-driven" feedback loop to increase supply. Doctors may recommend that you pump after each feeding, or at least
after some of them, to try to convince your body that you need more milk.
Our general knowledge of the biology of lactation suggests this could be
helpful, although I can find no research that gives any helpful guidance on
how to do this most successfully.

You'll also find a variety of suggestions on the internet about how to
increase your milk supply. These include herbal remedies—fenugreek is
the most common, although others, like nettle tea, do come up—as well as
particular foods (dark beer, for example) and a suggestion that you stay
hydrated.

It is always good to stay hydrated, but there is no reliable evidence that
it promotes milk production.[21] Beer actually makes things worse (more on
this on page 104).

The evidence on herbal remedies is mixed.[22] To take fenugreek as an
example, a 2016 review article covered two small randomized studies of
the effect of fenugreek consumption on breast milk. In one study, milk
production was increased. In the other, it was not. Evidence on other
herbal remedies (shatavari, malunggay) shows similarly mixed results.
None of these herbs shows any side effects at the recommended doses, so
it will not hurt you to try them, but they are not magic bullets.

There is more positive evidence on pharmaceutical remedies. In particular, the drug domperidone has been shown in a variety of randomized
studies to increase milk production.[23] (Unfortunately, it is not available in
the US, so this may be somewhat unhelpful to point out. Readers in the
UK can get it there, and it is also available in Canada.)

It is possible that no matter what you do, you will have little or no
milk—this isn't common, but it does happen, and it's often a surprise when
it does, since it is not frequently discussed. This is typically diagnosed as
insufficient glandular tissue (IGT), which simply means a lack of sufficient milk glands. For some women, this is a congenital condition—if this
is you, you'll likely have to supplement, at least to some extent.

Women who have had a breast reduction may also have a limited milk supply, depending on the method of reduction. Again, some degree of sup-plementation may be necessary.[24]

On the other side, you can have too much milk. This can happen natu-rally, or it can result from an overenthusiastic attempt to avoid the too-little-milk problem. The recommendation of adding pumping sessions after nursing sessions early on to increase milk supply can overcompensate—I know a few women who were zealous pumpers early on and then found themselves with liters of extra milk and very uncomfortable breasts.

The main problems with an oversupply are that it can be *very* uncom-fortable and can increase your risk of mastitis. Your breasts become en-gorged with milk; they are hard and hot, and they ache. Pumping can relieve the discomfort, but it contributes to the feedback loop and pro-longs the issue. If you want to calm down the supply, you have to deal with the engorgement problem.

There are a variety of recommended techniques to do this—acu-puncture, acupressure, particular kinds of massage, cold packs, hot packs, breast-shaped hot packs, cabbage leaves, and so on.[25] The evidence on these is spotty—there are a few randomized trials, most of which are small and subject to some bias. Cold and hot packs do seem to provide some re-lief, as do cold or room-temperature cabbage leaves. (Yes, you read that right: cabbage. You keep the leaves in the fridge and wrap your breasts in them. No one said being a mom was glamorous.)

One trial shows some benefit of something called *gua sha* therapy, which involves scraping the skin to produce light bruising. Gwyneth Pal-trow swears by this, so take what you will from that.

In addition to pain, an issue with oversupply is that when the baby does start to nurse, the milk may come very fast and overwhelm him, making it hard to actually eat. Basically, it is like you trying to drink from a firehose. Pumping for a couple of minutes—or hand-expressing milk—right before you nurse can help with this problem. It will also im-prove as the baby gets bigger and the oversupply problems calm down.

THE BREASTFEEDING DIET

"Hi Emily!" Humphrey wrote. "The baby is doing great. But Maggie's parents say she can't eat cauliflower or drink tap water because she is breastfeeding. They said the baby will cry more. Could this be right?"

After nine months of careful food avoidance, it adds insult to injury to think that breastfeeding will introduce a similar set of restrictions. Can you return to your rare steak? Those unpasteurized cheeses you've been craving—are they still off-limits? And what about a glass of wine—or even a couple of glasses? Is that okay?

Good news: mostly, breastfeeding moms have no dietary restrictions.

Let's start with the food part. The only food women are medically advised to avoid during breastfeeding is high-mercury fish.[26] That's it! No swordfish, king mackerel, tuna. But other fish are fine, as are unpasteurized cheeses, sushi, rare steak, deli meats, and on and on.

If your baby is suffering from colic—excessive crying as an infant—there is some evidence that avoiding common dietary allergens could help. For more on this, see page 35.

What about cauliflower?

There *is* something of an old wives' tale that gassy foods (cauliflower, broccoli, beans) lead to a gassy baby, and can make colic worse. I can find only one paper on this, and it is based on a mail survey that asked parents about many foods and compared the food consumption for babies with colic to those without.[27] Although this study did claim to find some minimal evidence that cauliflower and broccoli lead to more colic, the problems with the data collection and analysis are so significant (use of mail survey with poor response rate, excessive response among people who were hyperconcerned about breastfeeding, problems with statistical precision) that I think it is safe to ignore it.

Eat what you want.

What about alcohol? Many women hear—from the internet, typically not from their doctors—that they should avoid alcohol altogether, or that if they drink at all, they should "pump and dump." On the other side, some people will tell you that having alcohol (beer, specifically) will increase your milk supply. So you should have more! Are either of these true?

No, not really.[28]

When you drink, the alcohol level in your milk is about the same as your blood alcohol level. The baby consumes the milk, not the alcohol directly, so the level of alcohol they are exposed to is extremely low. One paper carefully calculates that even if you had *four* drinks very quickly and then breastfed at the maximum blood alcohol level, the baby would still be exposed to only a very, very low concentration of alcohol, one that is extremely unlikely to have any negative effects.[29] And this is in a kind of "worst-case scenario." This paper cautions that drinking four drinks quickly will impair your ability to parent and is not healthy, so it should be avoided, but the issue isn't alcohol in your breast milk. Therefore, *there is no need to pump and dump.* The milk has the same alcohol concentration as your blood. As that goes down, so does the milk alcohol level. It isn't stored in the milk.

Given this, it is not surprising that we do not find much evidence of the impact of a mother's alcohol consumption on her infant. There are some reports that babies sleep in shorter intervals when they consume milk after their mom has been drinking, but this isn't supported in all studies. And no long-term impacts have been identified.

What if you want to be super, super cautious and not expose your baby to alcohol *at all*? No problem. You can have a drink, but you need to wait for two hours afterward to let the alcohol metabolize before breastfeeding. For two drinks, that increases to four hours.[30]

These studies all caution—correctly—that we do not know much about binge drinking, or frequent heavy drinking (three or more drinks every day). Many women who binge drink frequently also did so during pregnancy, and they differ in other ways from women who do not binge drink. Even if you are not pregnant or nursing, binge drinking isn't good for your health. Binge drinking during pregnancy is very dangerous for your baby, and after birth, it will impair your ability to parent.

On the flip side, I'm sorry to report that drinking does not improve your milk supply. If anything, it may lessen it a bit, so if you are struggling with supply early on, do not consider alcohol as a supply booster.[31]

Along with alcohol, many women worry about the impact of taking medication while nursing. It's beyond the scope of this book to go through the interactions of every medication, but generally, most are safe and your doctor is a good source for more information. You can also search for virtually any drug in the LactMed database online.[32]

Two drug groups are common enough to deserve some discussion here: painkillers (i.e., those you'd use after birth) and antidepressants.

Childbirth is uncomfortable, and afterward, you'll likely be in significant pain for a few days or longer. The first line of defense is Tylenol or ibuprofen, typically (in the latter case) in quite high doses. These are well tolerated and fine for use while breastfeeding.

However, ibuprofen isn't always enough, especially for women who have had a C-section. Codeine used to be a common next step, but more recent data has suggested that exposure during breastfeeding has significant nervous system effects in babies; it makes them extremely sleepy, and in a few examples, there were thought to be severe consequences.[33] As a result, newer recommendations generally advise against prescribing codeine or other opioids like oxycodone.[34]

Having said this, the recovery from childbirth, especially a C-section, can be extremely challenging, so your doctor may prescribe opioids, with appropriate caution. If these drugs are prescribed, it is generally for a short time and at the lowest dose possible. The tension between pain relief and breastfeeding is one you'll need to work through with your doctor.

The news on antidepressants is considerably better. All antidepressants are secreted in breast milk, but there is little evidence of negative impacts on the baby. Postpartum depression is serious, and treatment is important. Although there are some differences in the extent to which different antidepressants pass into breast milk, it is generally accepted that women should be prescribed the drugs that work for them. If you have been on antidepressants before and know which one is effective for you, then that is what you should use.[35] If not, the first-line SSRIs for nursing mothers are paroxetine and sertraline, which transfer to breast milk at the lowest levels.

A final note is on caffeine. Most people find it's fine to have caffeine while nursing, and there is certainly no literature suggesting risks to the baby. However, some babies are quite sensitive to caffeine and get very fussy and irritable. If you find this is the case, you may have to avoid it.

Tap water, though? Go for it. Hydration is important for everyone, breastfeeding or not. Take the water anywhere you can get it.

PUMPING

A couple of years ago, MIT held a hack-a-thon to try to come up with better design ideas for a breast pump. Nothing marketable has yet come out of this, but we are all holding our breath, because breast pumps generally suck.

Here are some problems women have articulated: painful, difficult to use, requires constant cleaning, loud, heavy, ineffective. And these are just problems with the pump! Never mind the problems with actually having to do the pumping at work or while traveling—there is work time lost, and the endless problems of pumping in random airport bathrooms. Not to mention the TSA, who will carefully put their explosive-detecting wand over each bottle of milk you have lovingly packed up for the trip home.

I remember distinctly my joy at arriving in the Milwaukee airport and finding that they had a pumping pod—a little pod, with a lockable door, complete with an outlet and a seat. It is telling that this prompted a wildly excited call to Jesse and an ongoing fondness for Milwaukee (slogan: *Milwaukee: Genuine American*).

There have been some pumping innovations in the past few years. There is now a product called the Freemie, which is a pumping system where the cups effectively fit inside your bra and also collect the milk. The key, I think, is that the pump motor itself is quite small so you can store it in a pocket or clip it to your clothing. This postdates my nursing, and I could not get my friend Heidi to try it for research purposes, but I did hear from women who swear by it. In principle it allows you to, say, walk around outside while pumping. Someone told me she knows doctors who do surgery hooked up to this, but I think this falls in the realm of anecdote.

There are basically three reasons to use a breast pump. Let's review.

First, if you are struggling with low supply early on, your doctor may suggest you try pumping after some (or all) feedings to increase your supply. As noted earlier, the theory is good here, although there isn't much empirical evidence. If this is your only use of the pump, it may be a good idea to rent one from the hospital—it will be a better-quality pump. And you probably aren't going anywhere much at first.

Second, many women pump early on so they can start to give their baby the occasional bottle. Of course, you will pump while the kid gets the bottle, but if you want to have one ready for the first time, you'll have to pump beforehand. You may also want to do this to build up a supply of milk if you are planning to return to work.

I recall the logistics of this being complicated, especially when I was nursing Penelope and my supply was underwhelming. Some of the books told you to pump two hours after a feeding, even if the baby wasn't up, since then there would be some milk. But sometimes she wanted to eat right away when she woke up, and there wasn't much milk! Thinking back, these were among the most stressful moments of the early days.

There isn't really any scientific advice about this, so your best bet to limit stress may just be to have a concrete plan. Many women report that it works well to choose one feeding—likely in the morning, since that is when the milk is most plentiful—and just pump after that feeding. You'll get a bit of milk each time, and if you start early, over a week or two you'll get enough to give a bottle. Then while the kid has that bottle, you can pump another bottle during that feeding.

Finally, the main thing women use the pump for is to replace breast-feeding sessions after they're back at work. The idea is that you pump at approximately the same times the baby would eat, and they eat what you pump the next day. If you are a prolific pumper, you may pump enough extra to freeze.

There is no getting around this: most women find it difficult and unpleasant. Your job is supposed to provide breaks for pumping, but they may not always follow the rules. If you have your own office, super, but if not, pumping is often relegated to less than ideal locations. One doctor I spoke to said she pumped in the coed locker room, in full view of everyone (she used a towel to cover). Companies over a certain size are required to provide lactation rooms, but this isn't always followed, and there is no requirement that the rooms be nice.

Even in a perfect situation, you're supposed to wash the pump parts after every usage, and it just takes time. (Pumping wipes can help with this part.) If you pump for thirty minutes three times a day—not unusual at all—these are ninety minutes you could be doing something else.

It is possible to work while pumping—in some cases—and I strongly suggest you get a hands-free pumping bra. At a minimum you want to be able to read something on your phone. Many people suggest you try to relax, look at pictures of your baby, and generally wind down while pumping. The idea is that this will increase supply. There is no direct evidence for this; one study of moms pumping for babies in the NICU showed that being near their babies increased milk production, but this is pretty distant evidence.[36]

Oh, and while you are spending all your time hooked up to this pump, we should probably say that it's not as effective as your baby at milk removal. Even a really great pump doesn't replicate the baby. This varies across women—some women can have no problem fully breastfeeding but literally never get any milk from a pump; others find producing enough milk is no problem.

There is no perfect solution here. I had a good friend who had what seemed like a dream setup: her job was flexible and her kid's day care was next door, so she just popped over to nurse the baby a few times a day. It seemed amazing—until she tried to go away for a day and found her son wouldn't take a bottle.

We are all holding our breath for better pumping technology. MIT—get on this!

As a final note: For some women who struggle in an ongoing way with latching, pumping is the only option for the duration. This approach—where you only pump and never nurse—is called exclusive pumping (EP). If you find yourself in this situation, there is not much evidence to guide you on how to do it, but there are a lot of moms online who will help.

The Bottom Line

- Breastfeeding can be very hard!
- On early interventions:
  - Skin-to-skin contact early on can improve likelihood of breastfeeding success.
- On latching:
  - Nipple shields work for some women, although they can be hard to quit.
  - There is very limited evidence that fixing a tongue tie or lip tie can improve nursing.
- On pain:
  - Fixing a tongue tie can improve pain for Mom.
  - There isn't much evidence on how to fix nipple pain, but focusing on the latch may help.
  - If you are still in pain a few minutes into a feeding, or a few weeks into nursing, get help; it could be an infection, which would be treatable, or some other problem with a solution.
- On nipple confusion:
  - Not supported in the data.

continued ...

- On milk supply:
  - The majority of women will have their milk come in within three days after the baby's birth, but for about a quarter, it will take longer.
  - The biological feedback loop is compelling: nursing more should produce more supply.
  - Evidence on the effectiveness of non-drug remedies (e.g., fenugreek) on supply is limited.
- On pumping:
  - It sucks.

Sleep Position and Location

My children have a very old board book, a hand-me-down or tag sale purchase, called *Wynken, Blynken, and Nod.* At the end of the book, there is an illustration of a baby in his crib. What strikes me every time I see this image is just how much stuff there is in the crib with him. Stuffed toys, a blanket, crib bumpers, a pillow. My children's cribs—even when they were toddlers—contained nothing but a tiny security blanket and a water bottle. When we finally moved Penelope to a toddler bed at three years old, it took her months to figure out the concept of covers.

Parenting recommendations change over time, but perhaps nothing has changed more from our childhood to the current era than recommendations for sleep. When we were children, it wasn't uncommon for babies to be put to sleep on their stomachs, covered in a fuzzy blanket, in a crib surrounded by a bumper. You can see why this would make sense: babies are small, and cribs are not inherently cozy. There is something a little jarring about a tiny baby alone in a giant crib.

The latest recommendations from the American Academy of Pediatrics are starkly opposed to the toy-and-blanket-filled crib. The AAP says infants should sleep alone in a crib (or bassinet) and should be placed in the crib on their back to sleep. There should be nothing in the crib with the baby. Bumpers—pads that wrap around crib slats to prevent little hands or feet from getting stuck—should not be used. Infants should sleep in their own crib or bassinet—not in the parents' bed—although the crib or bassinet should be in the room with the parents.

These recommendations are broadly part of a safe sleep campaign designed to lower the risk of SIDS (which is now more accurately referred to as sudden unexpected infant death, or SUID, but given that most people are familiar with the acronym SIDS, I will stick with that here).

The initial part of this campaign, "Back to Sleep," focused on the importance of always putting infants to sleep on their backs. More recent additions have focused on co-sleeping and room sharing.

The AAP sleep recommendations are simple to understand, but many people find them difficult to follow, especially in the exhausted haze of new parenting when many of us would empty our bank account for two hours of uninterrupted sleep. Many infants sleep better on their stomachs, and the temptation to try this when nothing else has worked is powerful. Similarly, it can be tempting to keep the baby in bed with you, especially when you are breastfeeding. When your baby falls asleep while nursing and you know they will stay asleep if you keep them next to you, it's hard to move them.

On the opposite end, the instruction to keep the baby's bed in your room may be equally difficult. Jesse has never been able to sleep in the same room as the kids. When Finn was born, we had him in our room for a few weeks; Jesse slept on an air mattress in the unfinished attic. This did not feel like a long-term plan.

All of this makes these decisions both important and very hard. Thinking about them requires thinking carefully about risks.

SIDS, AND THINKING ABOUT RISK

Excluding birth defects, SIDS is the most common cause of death for full-term infants in the first year of life in the US. By definition, SIDS is the unexplained death of a seemingly healthy infant under a year old, and 90 percent of these deaths occur in the first four months of life.

The causes of SIDS are not well understood. It seems to occur when a baby spontaneously stops breathing and doesn't start again. It is more common in vulnerable infants—premature babies, for example—and in boys.

Among the most haunting aspects of parenting is the vulnerability that comes with having the thing you love most in the world be out of your control. There is no parent I know who doesn't, at least at times, have the instinct to keep their child at home, to never let them out of their sight, to literally never let go.

And yet we do take risks. We let our children learn to ride a bike—knowing that they'll get some skinned knees. We let them play with other children, knowing that at least some of the time, they'll return home with a nasty cold or the stomach flu. In these cases, it is not so hard to think about how to weigh the risks against the benefits. On one hand, stomach flu is yucky; on the other hand, playing with other kids is both fun and important for development. So we weigh them out, probably deciding it's fine for our children to play with other kids, but maybe not when those kids are actively sick.

It is much harder to think about risks when there is a possibility of a catastrophic outcome—serious illness or death.

The first step is to put sleep risks in the context of the risks that we are implicitly accepting every day. We put our children in the car, which is not perfectly safe. This isn't a danger we think about much, but it is there. On the scale of the underlying levels of risk we are implicitly accepting, some of the risks we talk about below—while real—are small.

Second, we have to recognize that sleep choices have real quality-of-life impacts. If co-sleeping is the only way you can get any sleep, then you may choose to do it to preserve your mental health, ability to drive, and ability to function overall—all things that also benefit your child. And these crucial choices may outweigh a very tiny risk, even a tiny risk of a terrible thing. It's easy to dismiss people who remind you to take care of yourself. But taking care of yourself is actually part of your responsibility.

It is not easy to even think about parenting choices associated with risk, let alone make them. In at least some cases here, the risks are clear and not vanishingly small; in those cases, the choice is easy. In others, it seems clear the risks are really not there at all. But in some of these cases—co-sleeping, in particular—more complex considerations come into play, and we'll need to confront them.

When I was writing this book, I talked to my friend Sophie, who co-slept with her youngest child for many months. Sophie is a highly trained doctor, and clearly not ignorant of the risks of co-sleeping. She told me she didn't make this decision lightly, and she didn't disagree with the AAP's guidelines. But co-sleeping was the only way her baby would sleep, so she took all the steps that have been shown to minimize the associated risks: she and her partner didn't smoke or drink, and they took all the covers and blankets off of the bed. Even with these precautions, she accepted the possibility of a small risk.

Ultimately, this is a choice parents have to make, and it's best to make it with full information. The medical recommendations to avoid SIDS have four components. Infants should be (1) on their back, (2) alone in the crib, (3) in their parents' room, and (4) with nothing soft around.

RECOMMENDATION 1:
"ON THEIR BACK"

Until the early 1990s, the most common sleeping position for infants—in the US and elsewhere—was on their stomach. The reason for this is likely that many infants sleep better this way—they don't wake up as much.[1]

However, as early as the 1970s, there were some clues that stomach sleeping was associated with a higher risk of SIDS.[2] Studies comparing populations with different sleeping patterns showed worse outcomes for the group that slept on their stomach.

These early studies were largely ignored, and through the mid-1980s, most pediatricians recommended that infants be put to sleep on their stomachs. The edition of *Dr. Spock's Baby and Child Care* that my parents used says, "I think it is preferable to accustom babies to sleep on the stomach from the start."[3]

This changed in the early 1990s with the release of a series of studies showing more directly that stomach sleeping was associated with a dramatically elevated risk of SIDS.

Studying this problem with data is challenging. SIDS deaths are thankfully rare, so some of the more standard research techniques are difficult to implement. Even a very large randomized trial or observational study is not likely to have enough observations to draw statistically meaningful conclusions.[4] Instead, researchers typically look at SIDS using case-control studies.

In 1990, the *British Medical Journal* published one of these studies, based on data drawn from the UK.[5] The researchers focused on a particular area (Avon) and identified sixty-seven infants in that area who had died of SIDS. They then searched for two control infants for each of the cases—those of similar age, or similar age and birth weight—and surveyed both sets of parents.

Their most striking findings related to stomach sleeping. Nearly all the infants who died of SIDS were sleeping on their stomachs (62 of the 67 infants, or 92 percent). However, among the surviving infants, only 56 percent were sleeping on their stomachs. Based on this comparison, the authors argued that babies who sleep on their stomachs are *eight times* as likely to die of SIDS. This paper also cited overheating as a risk factor—the babies who died were more likely to be wearing heavy clothing to bed, sleeping under a lot of bedding, or sleeping in a hot room.

Other research with similar approaches shows the same results.[6] This is not the only type of evidence we have. There is a biological mechanism for the link: babies tend to sleep more deeply on their stomachs, and SIDS risk is increased with deeper sleep. In addition, we have evidence from the Netherlands based on variation in sleep position over time.

In the 1970s, a Dutch campaign encouraged parents to put their children to sleep on their stomachs. In 1988, the recommendation changed, and parents were told to put children to sleep on their backs. With these changes in sleep position came changes in incidences of SIDS. SIDS rates rose after the stomach-sleep recommendation, and fell after parents were told to put their children to sleep on their backs.[7] Alone, this type of variation over time wouldn't prove a causal relationship between SIDS and sleep position. But combined with the other evidence, it begins to paint a causal picture.

By the early 1990s, it seemed clear that stomach sleeping was risky. A review article in the *Journal of the American Medical Association* at this time discussed all the evidence, and concluded that despite having no randomized trial, the data warranted a serious effort to prevent parents from putting their babies in this position to sleep.[8]

This effort came in the form of the aforementioned "Back to Sleep" campaign, which began in the US in 1992, and was remarkably successful. In surveys done in 1992, researchers found that around 70 percent of babies were put to sleep on their stomach.[9] By 1996, this figure was only 20 percent. This large change in sleeping position was also accompanied by a decrease in the SIDS rate, further suggesting that sleep position plays a role in SIDS.

The "Back to Sleep" campaign emphasizes the importance of putting an infant on their back, not on either their side or their stomach. The evidence, however, largely points to stomach sleeping as high risk, rather than side sleeping. The concern about side sleeping is mainly that infants can inadvertently roll onto their stomach. The back sleeping recommendations are, therefore, really designed to avoid the risk of stomach sleeping as fully as possible.

One note: If your infant does roll over, there is no need to go rolling them back. Once they can do this on their own, the highest risk of SIDS has also passed, probably because the baby now has enough head strength to move their head to breathe more easily.

Side Effects: Deformational Plagiocephaly

There is one substantial side effect to back sleeping: deformational plagiocephaly, or, colloquially, flat head. Infants who sleep on their back are at higher risk for head flattening. The frequency of this issue has been rising over time since the implementation of "Back to Sleep."[10]

Deformational plagiocephaly is more likely to occur if the infant always has their head turned to one particular side when they sleep. And at least some literature suggests it is exacerbated by having some degree of head flattening at birth.[11] It is also more common in twins and premature babies. It doesn't have any effect on brain growth or function, so this is purely an aesthetic concern. Making sure your baby has tummy time during the day or, generally, does not spend all day lying on their back can help avoid this condition.

Flat head is at least somewhat fixable. The standard treatment is a helmet, which is worn for most of the day and night, but there is some debate over whether the helmet actually fixes the problem more successfully than doing nothing. If you face this issue, discuss your treatment options with your pediatrician.[12]

RECOMMENDATION 2: "ALONE IN THE CRIB"

The second piece of advice from the AAP is to have your infant alone in their crib. In other words, no co-sleeping.

This recommendation is extremely controversial among parents.

Some people strongly support co-sleeping. A common argument from this group is that this is how infants have slept for millennia. This is true: there was no crib in the cave, and even now it is common for infants and children in many cultures to sleep in bed with their parents for many years. This is, however, not a reliable argument for safety. There are plenty of ways we have changed infant practices to improve survival.

A common argument in the other direction is that there have been infant deaths from suffocation under a sleeping parent. This is also true. But the fact that this is a possibility doesn't mean the risk is large, and the risk may be mitigated by how you co-sleep.

The real question, then, is whether the risk of SIDS is significantly higher when co-sleeping, and if so, how large the increase is. Evidence on this comes, again, from case-control studies similar to those used to study the role of sleep position. In this case, researchers collect information about a set of infant deaths, focusing on the usual sleep location of the infant, where they were sleeping when they died, and whether they were breastfed or bottle-fed, as well as on characteristics of the parents, including their typical alcohol consumption and smoking habits. The researchers then find a set of controls—infants similar in terms of age and other characteristics, but who survived. They ask the parents the same questions and compare their answers.

Many of the individual studies of this are small, so it is helpful to have "meta-analyses," which combine data from many similar studies. One excellent example was published in the *British Medical Journal* in 2013.[13] This paper combines data from studies run in Scotland, New Zealand, Germany, and elsewhere (although notably not the US). What is helpful about this analysis is that the authors explicitly tried to estimate the excess risk in groups with varying behaviors. They focused on whether the parents smoked or used alcohol (more than two drinks a day), and whether the infant was breastfed.

The following graph—based on results from their paper—shows differences in death rates for infants who do and do not bed share. The absolute risks here are constructed based on a normal-weight, nonpremature infant. The various bars show different combinations of risk factors.

The first thing this graph makes clear is that both overall SIDS rates

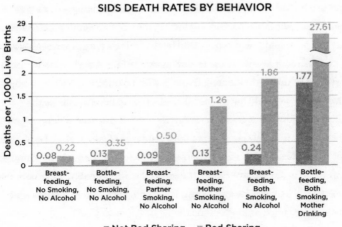

SIDS DEATH RATES BY BEHAVIOR

and the increased risks from co-sleeping are much larger in the presence of other risk factors—parental smoking and drinking, in particular. In the most extreme example, the predicted mortality for a bottle-fed infant with parents who both smoke and where the mother drinks more than two drinks a day is 27 deaths per 1,000 births, fully 16 times higher than the comparable infant who doesn't share the parents' bed.

The observation that smoking, in particular, increases the risks associated with bed sharing is widely shared in other literature.[14] The mechanisms for links between SIDS and smoking are not fully understood but seem to relate to the role of chemicals in secondhand smoke and their interference with infant breathing. This problem becomes more acute if the baby is closer to the smoker (even if the parent is not actively smoking).[15]

This graph also speaks to perhaps the more central question for many families, which is, are there still risks to co-sleeping if you do it as safely as possible—that is, if neither parent smokes or drinks a lot, and if the baby is breastfed?

The data here says yes. The risk of death for infants who do not bed share in the lowest risk group is 0.08 SIDS deaths per 1,000 births. For those who bed share, it is 0.22 deaths per 1,000 births. Again, we want to put these risks into a broader context. In the US, the overall infant mortality rate is around 5 deaths per 1,000 births. This therefore represents a very small increase relative to the overall mortality rate. A perhaps more useful way to say this is that among families with no other risk factors, roughly 7,100 of them would have to avoid co-sleeping to prevent one death.

The finding that co-sleeping carries a small risk even if done as safely as possible is largely consistent across studies, and although the exact size of the increased risk varies from report to report, they are in a similar range.[16] These risks are concentrated early in life. Notably, there does not seem to be any elevated risk from co-sleeping after three months *if* both parents are not drinking or smoking.

Putting these risk analyses together, a main takeaway here is that if you are going to co-sleep, you should definitely not drink a lot or smoke, and neither should your partner. Limiting these behaviors will let you co-sleep in the safest way possible, although it will not completely eliminate the risks. On the other side, though, there may be some benefits.

The main benefit—the one I see cited by moms most often—is that bed sharing is convenient, and if you try to move an infant who has fallen asleep, they tend to wake up. This is certainly true, at least for some babies, and probably something you can evaluate yourself. If the baby wakes up less, parents may also sleep more.

Indeed, for my friend Sophie—and other friends, many of them doctors, who told me they co-slept—more sleep was the main reason to do it. For Sophie, whose family comprised two working parents and two other children, it didn't seem feasible for her to be up all night going back and forth to a crib. Never mind that her son also slept much better in her bed than out of it. It came down to co-sleep or no sleep, and Sophie and her husband ultimately decided that having the baby in their bed was the best thing for their whole family.

A second possible benefit, one that we can evaluate with data, is the possibility of improved success with breastfeeding. Certainly, there is a correlation: moms who bed share are also more likely to be breastfeeding and to persist until the child is older.[17] But this doesn't necessarily point to causality. We know from data that women who have a strong desire to breastfeed before they give birth are more likely to bed share.[18] It could be that the desire to breastfeed prompts bed sharing, not the other way around. And indeed, the one randomized trial that evaluated the relationship between breastfeeding and having an infant in an attached cot rather than a separate bed fails to find any link between bed sharing and breastfeeding.[19]

This doesn't mean there are no benefits for your family to bed sharing, just that it probably isn't a panacea to improve your breastfeeding success.

RECOMMENDATION 3: "IN THE PARENTS' ROOM"

In the spate of recommendations, bed sharing is forbidden, but room sharing is encouraged. The American Academy of Pediatrics recommends that infants be in their parents' room through at least the first six months, and ideally the first year, of life as a guard against SIDS. The theory is that parents can be more attentive to the baby if they are in the same room.

The evidence on room sharing and SIDS is substantially less complete than the evidence on bed sharing. The studies have the same basic structure, but they are smaller and there are fewer of them. Less attention is paid to other factors that might influence the relationship. For example, what if you have a video monitor in the baby's room? Is that enough? You will not find evidence for that here.

With that caveat, we can review the studies we *do* have.

To take one concrete example, consider a study published in the *British Medical Journal* in 1999. The authors, using a sample of about 320 infant deaths and 1,300 control infants, argue that sleeping in a room alone is associated with a higher risk of death.[20] However, the results in the paper are inconsistent. For example, it matters a lot whether they analyze the usual sleeping location or the most recent sleeping location; there seems to be no risk when they analyze usual sleeping location, but a higher risk when they analyze the most recent one. It's not clear why this would be, and leads to concerns that something else unusual happened on the last night of life.

In forming their recommendations on room sharing, the AAP cited this study and three others.[21] These show similarly small increases in SIDS rates for babies who sleep in their own room, but the results are not overwhelming. They all tend to be very sensitive to which variables researchers adjust for, and, important, most of these studies were not actually designed to look at room sharing. Although these studies are too small to really analyze mitigating factors, the benefits of room sharing seem to be larger if the infant also sleeps on their stomach[22] and depend on whether parents also sometimes bed share.[23]

While I think one can debate the merits of room sharing at all, given the data, in my view, the AAP's recommendation that room sharing extend through the baby's first year is problematic.

Why do I say this?

The vast majority—up to 90 percent—of SIDS deaths occur in the first four months of life, so sleeping choices after four months are very unlikely to matter for SIDS. This also shows up in the data. The choice of sharing a room, or even sharing a bed, does not seem to affect SIDS risk after three or four months, at least for parents who are nonsmokers.[24]

This means there is seemingly no benefit to extending room sharing for so long. There is, however, a real cost: child sleep. In a 2017 study, researchers evaluated whether a child's sleeping in a room with a parent made for worse sleep. They found that it did. At four months old, total sleep time was similar for babies sleeping in a parents' room and those sleeping in their own room, but sleep was more consolidated (i.e., in longer stretches) for those in the latter group. This makes sense: their own room will be quieter.

At nine months, infants who slept alone slept longer; this effect was largest for those who slept alone by four months, but also appears for babies who moved to their own room between four and nine months. Most notably, these differences were still present when the child was two and a half years old: children who slept alone by nine months slept forty-five minutes more during the night than those who were room sharing at nine months. Sleep is crucial for child brain development; it is not just a selfish parental indulgence. Of course, this may not be causal—maybe parents move their kids to their own room when they start sleeping well—but it is suggestive.

Related to this, it should be said that if you plan to sleep train your child, success is very unlikely while the child is sleeping in your room. And finally, most people sleep better without a child in the room, and parents being well rested is important, too.

Pulling all this together, I believe the AAP recommendations go too far. If you want to share a room with your child, by all means do. And perhaps—*perhaps*—the data warrants a mild recommendation in favor of very early room sharing. But to tell people they need to keep their child in their room for a year, sacrificing both short- and long-term sleep success with no clear benefit in the process, may not be a good policy.

The Sofa

Across virtually all studies of sleep location, the one thing that jumps out as really, really risky is babies sharing a sofa with an adult. Death rates as a result of this behavior are twenty to sixty times higher than the baseline risk. It is not difficult to see why: an exhausted adult falls asleep holding an infant on a cushiony sofa, and it is easy for the infant to be smothered by a pillow. The unfortunate thing is that in at least some of these sofa deaths, the parent involved is trying to avoid the risks associated with bed sharing. They hope that if they sit up, they will stay awake, and then they fall asleep by accident. Even with the small risks of bed sharing, you'd be much better off sharing a bed than accidentally co-sleeping on a sofa.

RECOMMENDATION 4: "NO SOFT STUFF"

The final AAP guideline for sleep is that (aside from the baby) your child's crib should be empty, with no toys, no bumpers, no blankets or pillows. Nothing.

This is probably the easiest recommendation to follow. Other than adorableness, there is no reason to have toys or pillows in the baby's crib (bumpers may be a different story). There are also some advantages to this if you ever travel with your child. No parent wants to be carting along Lamby *and* Special Bear *and* Stinky Dino *and* Captain Poodle-pants when they travel to Grandma's house. If you can limit the number of things your child absolutely needs to fall asleep, your luggage will thank you.

In terms of risks, there are two central parts of the no-stuff-in-the-crib recommendation. One is that infants should not have blankets. This conclusion is based on the results of a number of the studies discussed previously. Infants who die of SIDS are more likely to be found with blankets over their heads than control infants. The infant-clothing industry has come up with a solution to this, which is the "wearable blanket"—basically, a zipped-up bag you put your child in. Since there is no real reason to have another kind of blanket, this recommendation seems like a reasonable one to follow.

The second part of the recommendation regards crib bumpers, which are forbidden by the AAP. In fact, some cities (Chicago, for example) have disallowed the sale of bumpers. The concern is that these can cause suffocation.

This recommendation is slightly more complicated since, in fact, there is a purpose for bumpers in the first place: without them, your child can get their arms and legs stuck between the crib rails. This is unlikely to be life-threatening, but can certainly hurt the baby.

It is useful to think about the magnitude of the bumper risk. A 2016 paper in the *Journal of Pediatrics* counted all the US deaths attributed to bumpers between 1985 and 2012.[25] They found forty-eight. To put this in context, during this period there were about 108 million children born in the US and somewhere in the range of 650,000 total infant deaths. Eliminating bumpers in this period would therefore be expected to lower the risk of death by about 0.007 percent, preventing 1 in 13,500 deaths. By contrast, estimates suggest the "Back to Sleep" campaign reduced death risk by about 8 percent—preventing about 1 in 13 deaths. In other words, eliminating bumpers would have, at most, a very, very small effect on risk.

Does this mean you should have bumpers? No, not necessarily. Among other things, older children can use the bumpers to escape the crib and fall out, which can be dangerous on its own. This is just to say that the overall risk associated with them is small.

MAKING CHOICES

Armed with the data, we are now back to where we started in this chapter: thinking about risks, including the risks of terrible outcomes that we are afraid to contemplate. And yet we do need to think about them, and to think about them in the context of the size of the effects, and of what works for our individual families.

Looking back at the results above, it seems clear, first, that having your child sleep on their back and avoiding blankets and pillows and other soft items in the crib are good ideas. Avoiding sofa sleeping is also strongly recommended. These recommendations have the most compelling evidence, and are also the easiest to implement.

It also seems clear that smoking raises the risk of SIDS, especially if you choose to bed share.

Finally, looking at the data, we have to conclude that in terms of SIDS risk, choices about sleep location—in your bed, in your room—matter much more in the first four months of your baby's life.

This leaves us with a set of choices in the first few months of life—whether to share the bed, share the room but not the bed, or share neither. And since the data suggests that there is some risk to sharing the bed, and possibly also to having your child sleep in their own room, we may conclude the absolute safest thing is to have your child sleep in your room in their own bed for these first few months.

Yet this setup may not work for your family. Let's imagine that your preference is to share your bed with your infant—maybe you think it will be easier to breastfeed, or you simply want to have the baby close.

If this is the case, there is a strong temptation to dismiss the evidence on risk. It is easy to find parenting sources that point to one study that doesn't show significant impacts of bed sharing and say it proves there is no risk. This is not a rational way to make this decision. If you want to do this right, you need to confront the idea of risk, think about how to make it smaller (if you can), and then think about whether the (minimized) risk is one you are willing to take.

If you are going to bed share, start by making sure you are not smoking or drinking and that your bed is not full of covers and pillows. And think about your infant: if your baby was premature or had low birth weight, the baseline risk of SIDS is higher, and the absolute increase in risk from bed sharing will be higher also.

And then, finally, you want to really try to think about the numbers.

If we look at the main graph on page 119, and imagine that you have a full-term infant and are a breastfeeding mom who does not smoke or drink (and your partner doesn't, either), the evidence suggests that bed sharing increases the risk of death by 0.14 per 1,000 births. The death rate from car accidents in the first year of life is around 0.2 per 1,000 live births. The bed-sharing risk is therefore a real one, but it is smaller than some of the risks you are likely taking regularly.

With my own children, bed sharing wasn't appealing, but neither was room sharing. My daughter was in her own room immediately, and my son after a couple of weeks. We did everything we could to limit the risks to this—the crib was bare, we had a video monitor—but, knowing that sharing a room with an infant was not going to work for our family, we accepted the possibility of some increased risk.

This is not the choice everyone will make, but the bottom line is that it *is* a choice. If you do want to bed share, or don't want to room share, you can make this decision by thinking that the benefits for your whole family outweigh the risks, even if you accept there are some risks.

The Bottom Line

- There is good evidence that infants who sleep on their back are at lower risk for SIDS.
- There is moderate evidence that bed sharing is risky.
  - These risks are much higher if you or your partner smokes or drinks alcohol.
- There is some less-good evidence that room sharing is beneficial.
  - The benefits to room sharing die out in the first few months.
  - Infant and child sleep may be better if your child sleeps alone after the first few months.
- In the crib:
  - Wearable blanket: check!
  - Bumpers: very small risk, although small benefits as well.
- Sleeping on a sofa with an infant is extremely dangerous.

Organize Your Baby

When you're pregnant, especially for the first time, people have a lot of advice for you. One thing I recall vividly is another economist earnestly explaining to me that it is very important to get your child on a schedule *immediately* upon arriving home from the hospital. You should decide when they will eat and sleep, and impose that. Babies love it! (So he said.)

My fellow economist was not alone in this belief. A whole army of books and philosophies—Babywise being perhaps the most well-known—suggest getting your baby on a schedule right away. These recommend that, even very early on, when it really is very hard to predict when your baby will sleep, you attempt to impose structure, the idea being that the baby will adapt to and adopt the structure. This can be quite appealing to the new parent struggling to figure out how to understand their baby. Not to mention the promise that such a schedule would let parents better predict when they themselves can sleep.

We didn't listen to our fellow economist, and with Penelope, there was no schedule. When I was first pregnant with Finn, Jesse sent me the following transcript of a Messenger exchange from when Penelope was four weeks old.

> **oster.emily(23:41:00 (UTC)):** do you want to do something?
> **oster.emily(23:41:02 (UTC)):** I dont know what
> **oster.emily(23:41:06 (UTC)):** also, maybe we should have dinner sometime?
> **oster.emily(23:42:08 (UTC)):** hello?

Note that these messages were sent at midnight. Not only was Penelope not on a schedule, but neither, it seems, were we.

Eventually, of course, she did end up on a schedule, one that looked very much like all the other kids': sleep at night, three naps during the day at first, then two, then one, then finally none. But each of these transitions was a struggle—to implement, yes, but even just to figure out the timing of. How do you know when your child is ready to drop one of the naps? At some point when we were dropping the morning nap, our nanny went into the other room during lunch, and returned three minutes later to find Penelope asleep in her food.

And this isn't just about convenience or planning your day. Sleep is important! It's important for baby development, and for parents. Your child will be in a better mood if they get the right amount of sleep. For a toddler, napping too much may make it harder to get to sleep at night. This means no sleep for parents. If they nap too little, they may be too overtired to get to sleep at night. This also means no sleep for parents.

How much sleep is enough, and when should it happen? It seems like a simple question, but answers differ widely. Take, for example, the two category-killer sleep books: Ferber (*Solve Your Child's Sleep Problems*) and Weissbluth (*Healthy Sleep Habits, Happy Child*). Both provide some guidance on the amount you should expect your child to sleep.

The trouble is, they do not agree.

Ferber, for instance, says that at six months, a baby should sleep a total of about 13 hours: 9.25 hours at night, and two 1- to 2-hour naps. Weissbluth suggests this same six-month-old should sleep a total of about 14 hours, but with more of those hours falling at night: 12 hours at night, and two 1-hour naps. This is a 3-hour difference in the suggested nighttime sleep.

Weissbluth goes further, suggesting that if your child does not sleep much—for example, if they sleep only nine hours at night—this is a serious problem. And I quote: "Children who slept less not only tended to be more socially demanding, bratty, and fussy but they also behaved somewhat like hyperactive children. Later, I will explain how these fatigued, fussy brats are also more likely to become fat kids."[1] So, no pressure!

But note that nine hours of sleep at night is what Ferber recommends. So is this optimal sleep, or the path to obesity?

In addition, the age ranges for the various important transitions are wide and can be vague. The books generally note that around six weeks, infants start to sleep longer at night; at three to four months, naps start to consolidate; at around nine months, the third nap disappears; at a year to twenty-one months, the second nap disappears; and at three to four years, the final nap disappears. On these latter two transitions in particular, these ranges are wide. A year to twenty-one months is a long time!

Roughly speaking, these claims are based on averages across the population. To see this, consider a meta-analysis of studies of sleep duration.[2] The two graphs that follow show, based on this analysis, the expected length of the longest sleep period (which is almost always at night) and the number of naps, both graphed against age.

You can see general patterns emerging here. Around two months, there is a big jump up in the average longest sleep period—this is the consolidation of nighttime sleep. This then increases more slowly as the child ages.

The nap graph contains even more information. Nine to ten months is the point at which the average number of naps is two; at eighteen to twenty-three months, it moves all the way to one.

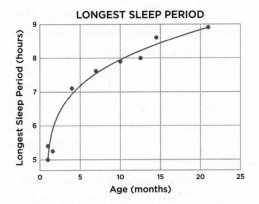

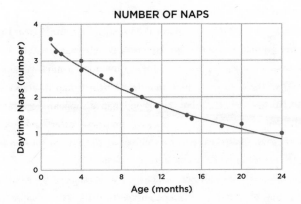

This paper also summarizes total sleep duration; newborns sleep an average of sixteen hours a day, which falls to thirteen or fourteen hours around one year.

This gives you a sense of what to expect if your child is the average child. Of course, your child is probably not exactly average, and these graphs fail to summarize variation across children.

One of the biggest innovations in data collection over the past few years is the ability to collect data through apps. The era of smartphone parenting has put data collection into overdrive for many of us, and sleep data is no exception. It is not surprising, therefore, to find researchers mining this data trove. One of the advantages of having *so much data* is that you can look at variations across people.

In 2016, five authors published a paper in the *Journal of Sleep Research* that used data from a Johnson & Johnson–sponsored app that allows parents to record infant sleep patterns.[3] They focused on the set of people who seemed to record reliably, and were able to isolate data from 841 children over a period of 156,989 sleep sessions. (This means the average parent in the study using the app is recording almost *two hundred* sleep sessions. That is devotion to data.) The granularity of the data allows for interesting analyses and, most important, for us to see how sleep varies across kids.

It varies a lot.

Take, as an example, the question of nighttime sleep length. In this data, the average six-month-old baby sleeps ten hours a night. Great—that's about what we saw in the studies I mentioned earlier. What about the baby at the 25th percentile (this would be a baby who didn't sleep much)? Nine hours. What about the 75th percentile? Eleven hours.

Now, what about the *whole* range of the data for six-month-olds? It turns out, in the data they see babies who sleep as few as six hours at night, and babies who sleep as many as fifteen hours.

This makes things a bit clearer: at least part of the reason the books are vague is that there is not really one answer to the question of how much children sleep at night.

Data on daytime sleep shows a similar amount of variation. The longest sleep session during the day on average increases from an hour to about two hours over the first two years of life, but there is a huge range in this, with some children napping not at all at most ages, and some for up to three hours at a stretch.

And similarly, the timing of the move from two naps to one also shows a lot of variation. Around eleven months, most children have two distinct naps, and by nineteen to twenty months most have one, but there is a long period of transition in the data, showing that the age at which children switch to a single nap varies quite widely.

In conclusion, many aspects of scheduling will be kid specific, and attempts to organize your baby are likely to meet with some of these variations. But not *everything* varies. In particular, one thing that doesn't show as much variation is wake-up times. Even at around five or six months, the majority of children wake between six and eight a.m. By the time they get to age two, the range is smaller—six thirty to seven thirty a.m.

Putting together the variation in total nighttime sleep and the lack of variation in wake-up time, you can naturally conclude that bedtimes vary a lot. They do. If you think your child needs a lot of sleep, you probably have to put them to bed earlier, since you cannot really get them to wake up later. If you try to schedule your child to go to bed late and sleep late into the morning, you will probably not succeed.

Some things about a second child are harder, the main one being the presence of the first child. But some things are easier, and at least in my experience, schedule is one of them. Before you have any children, you're on an adult schedule—wake up for work, eat dinner late, maybe stay up to watch some TV. Catch up on sleep on the weekends. Sometimes, maybe, you go to bed earlier, sometimes later.

Once you have even one child, you're on their schedule. Wake up between six thirty and seven thirty a.m., breakfast, nap, lunch, nap, dinner, bedtime around seven thirty p.m. (ideally). When the second child arrives, they are not on this schedule immediately, of course, but you know where you are going. The Messenger chat Jesse sent was intended as a warning about where we were headed, but we didn't get there at all. Yes, Finn was up during the night, but I was in bed with him—or, rather, with him in the cot next to me—from day one. We stuck to the schedule we'd used with Penelope, and he actually got there much faster than she did.

The other thing you realize with your second child is that the unscheduled mess of the first year does end. Your baby will, eventually, arrive at a more predictable sleep schedule. Maybe not right away, maybe not exactly the one you envisioned, but they will get there. And this is perhaps the most reassuring thing of all.

The Bottom Line

- There are some broad guidelines for sleep schedule.
  - Longer nighttime sleep develops around two months.
  - Move to three regular naps around four months.
  - Move to two regular naps around nine months.
  - Move to one regular nap around fifteen to eighteen months.
  - Drop napping around age three.
- There is tremendous variability across children, which you mostly cannot control.
- The most consistent schedule feature is wake-up time between six and eight a.m.
- Earlier bedtime = longer sleep.

Vaccination:
Yes, Please

In the 1950s, about five hundred people—mostly children—died of measles each year in the US; 3 to 4 million were sickened. In 2016, zero children in the US died of measles, and there were an estimated eighty-six cases.[1]

There is a very simple reason for this decline: the development of a measles vaccine.

Vaccinations are among the most significant public health triumphs of the past hundred years (public sanitation is another good one, although less controversial). Simply put, millions of lives worldwide have been saved by the introduction of vaccines for diseases like whooping cough, measles, smallpox, and polio. A tremendous amount of discomfort and itching, and also some deaths, have been prevented by the chicken pox vaccine. The vaccine for hepatitis B has reduced liver cancer. Newer vaccines also matter: the HPV vaccine has the potential to significantly lower rates of cervical cancer.

Despite this, vaccinations remain one of the most central focal points in the Mommy Wars. Some parents do not want their children vaccinated, fearing injury, autism, or some other unspecified downside. Some parents want to delay vaccines, feeling that risks will be mitigated by spacing out vaccinations.

These concerns—which have grown over time—have visible impacts on disease outbreaks. In May 2017, for example, there was a measles outbreak in Minnesota, with at least fifty cases. The outbreak was concentrated in the Somali immigrant community, where antivaccination activists had made efforts to convince the population that vaccines were linked to autism. Many families did not plan to vaccinate, or were waiting until their children were older. In the meantime, their children got measles.

A surprising aspect of vaccine resistance is that it tends to be stronger in areas with more educated parents. For most health outcomes—heart disease, obesity, diabetes—more educated people tend to be healthier. But in the case of vaccines, the correlation often goes the other way. Areas with more educated parents actually have, on average, *lower* vaccination rates.[2] This suggests it is not necessarily lack of information getting in the way of choosing vaccination.

The scientific consensus on vaccinations is extremely clear: vaccines are safe and effective. This conclusion is supported by a very wide range of doctors and medical organizations, and by government and non-government entities. But despite this, there are parents who choose not to vaccinate, and many of them are well educated and have thought about the decision. It is worth, therefore, at least visiting the evidence.

BACKGROUND

There have always been people who distrusted vaccines. A colleague of mine at Brown, Prerna Singh, studies resistance to vaccination—in this case, for smallpox—in China and India when the vaccine was first introduced. In that context, the concerns were focused on the harm the vaccine might cause, and the feeling that they might not prevent the disease anyway.

The most well-known concerns about vaccines at the moment relate to a possible link with autism, but there is an earlier round of vaccine-danger concerns dating from the 1970s. During this period, a series of case reports suggested that the pertussis vaccine—which prevents whooping cough and is given as part of the DTaP vaccine—might be linked to infant brain injury. It was subsequently revealed that this link was not supported in the data, but in the wake of the initial suggestion, there was a round of lawsuits filed against vaccine manufacturers.

The threat of these lawsuits was sufficient to almost completely shut down production of this vaccine. Vaccine prices rose and availability tanked. Lack of access to the vaccine presented a significant public health risk. In 1986, in response to this, Congress passed the National Childhood Vaccine Injury Act, which protected companies from being sued over mandated vaccinations. People who claim to be injured by vaccines can appeal to the federal government for compensation, but they cannot seek damages from the vaccine manufacturer.

A somewhat unfortunate side effect of this (sensible) policy solution is that it seems to imply that vaccine injuries are a real and substantial risk. (It might have been better to name the policy something else.) In practice, lawsuits brought by people reacting to flawed research were the motivation for the passage of the act, not any actual risks posed by vaccines. This policy is still in effect, and it unfortunately gives some background support to contemporary claims that vaccines are risky.

The latest round of vaccine resistance was tipped off by a former doctor ("former," since he subsequently lost his license) named Andrew Wakefield.[3] In 1998, Wakefield published a paper in the *Lancet*—a highly regarded medical journal—that suggested a link between autism and vaccines.[4] The paper is a summary of twelve case studies. The twelve children studied all had autism, and the paper claimed that in at least eight—and possibly more—of the twelve cases, the symptoms of autism began more or less immediately after the child received the measles, mumps, and rubella (MMR) vaccine.

Wakefield provided a hypothesized mechanism linking the two, related to digestive health.

First point: The conclusion of this paper is wrong. Other evidence, better evidence, from both before and after this article was published refutes this link. I review some of this in the following pages. Indeed, a vague case study of twelve children is hardly strong evidence in the first place, so it's not surprising that it didn't hold up.

But it turns out that the paper was also fraudulent. The children included in the sample were not—as Wakefield stated—all the kids who could have been included. Wakefield specifically chose children who supported his conclusion. In addition, many of the facts of the particular cases were falsified. Details were changed to make the onset of autism symptoms seem closer in time to the vaccinations. When, in reality, the onset of symptoms was six months or more after the vaccine, the reported case details suggested it was within a week or two.

Why would Wakefield do this? It turns out he was planning a lawsuit against vaccine manufacturers, and this would be part of the evidence. His motivation was the oldest reason in the book: money.

In 2010 the *Lancet* retracted the article, and Wakefield was stripped of his medical license. But the damage was done and Wakefield has never admitted the article was fraudulent or apologized. He continues to travel the world, hawking his discredited theories. The Somali immigrant community with the measles outbreak? They had had two visits from Wakefield over the preceding years.

Among the most insidious aspects of this episode is that it revived general concerns that vaccines are unsafe. Some people do not believe the link with autism, but still feel that vaccines may cause some other kind of injury. Antivaccination websites cite concerns about, for example, aluminum in vaccines, and also the general feeling that activating the immune system can cause brain injury.

These antivaccination websites seem evidence based; they cite papers and studies to support their position. On the other side, organizations like the Centers for Disease Control and the American Academy of Pediatrics assure people that vaccination is safe. A downside of their approach, however, is that they rarely confront the antivaccination literature head-on. There is little effort to explain why the papers cited on antivaccination websites are problematic (if they are). It can end up seeming like the anti-vaccination side is serious and evidence based, and the pro-vaccine side is just dismissively insisting you trust them.

This is not the case. The recommendations of the AAP, among others, are based on careful and complete evaluation of all the possible risks of vaccination.

VACCINE SAFETY

In 2011 the Institute of Medicine (IOM) published a nine-hundred-page tome entitled *Adverse Effects of Vaccines: Evidence and Causality.*[5] (I know what you're thinking: beach reading!)

The book is the product of years of work from a large number of re-searchers and practitioners. They were tasked with a daunting job: to evaluate the evidence for linkages between common vaccinations and a very large set of possible "adverse events."

They evaluated the evidence—from more than twelve thousand papers—on 158 vaccine-adverse event combinations. What does this mean? For each vaccine, the authors looked for evidence on a possible link between that particular vaccine and any claimed risk. The risks here are referred to as *adverse events.* So the authors looked for, say, evidence on a link between the MMR vaccine and seizures.[6]

What kind of evidence did they look for?

First, there are adverse-event reports: the CDC collates all reports of adverse events that people (parents, doctors, etc.) attribute to vaccination. You can explore this yourself online: searching for reports of links between MMR vaccine and autism yields a large number of reports from parents who claim their child developed autistic symptoms shortly after receiving the vaccine. You might have the instinct that these reports are enough to at least prove some link between vaccination and the outcome—but evidence of this type is tenuous at best.

Consider the following: Imagine that people believed that cutting an infant's fingernails was medically dangerous—that it led to illness or other complications. And imagine we set up an adverse-event reporting system for fingernail cutting.

In all likelihood, you'd get all kinds of reports. There would be parents saying that the day after they cut their infant's fingernails, the baby came down with a terrible fever. Others would say they had a very liquid-looking poop. You'd get reports of children who didn't sleep well for days after the fingernail cutting, and others about babies crying uncontrollably for hours.

These would all be true things that happened. But they would not be causally linked to the fingernail cutting! Sometimes infants get a fever; sometimes they have weird poops. Most babies do not sleep, and others cry a lot. In order to figure out whether there was any real link, you'd need to know the general base rate of these events—how likely people are to report them when there was no fingernail cutting. But that isn't something we have a reporting system for. There is no website where you can report every time your kid has an unusual poop.

You'd have to try to piece together whether these adverse events really seem more common among babies whose nails are cut than those whose aren't. This is especially hard for things that happen all the time, like "baby cried."

In your fingernail-reporting system, you probably *would* also learn something. You'd get a lot of reports of finger injury—cuts in need of Band-Aids. This is *not* something that happens all the time, and there is an obvious mechanism for the connection with nail cutting. So you would probably conclude that fingernail cutting is linked to accidental finger cutting, which is true (Penelope is at least one case report).

But how do we know the finger cutting is a real effect and the fever is not? How can we use evidence like this?

In the IOM report, the authors used reports like this in combination with evidence on mechanisms. Is there a biological reason to think this relationship would exist? In some cases, the biological link was so plausible that researchers drew conclusions based only on these adverse-event reports. In others, without a mechanism, they required more evidence to draw conclusions.

The second major piece of evidence comes from "epidemiological studies," which, in this case, compare children who are vaccinated with those who are not. These are typically not randomized, but they can be very large. If the adverse events reported are backed up by relationships in the population overall, this may support a link, even if the mechanism is not obvious.

The authors of this report classified each of their 158 possible links into one of four categories: convincingly supports (there is a convincing causal relationship between the vaccine and the event), favors acceptance (there is probably a causal relationship), favors rejection (unlikely, based on the available evidence), or insufficient evidence.

For the vast majority of these links, the evidence is insufficient. This includes things like the link between the MMR vaccine and multiple sclerosis onset, or between DTaP vaccines and SIDS. In these cases, the authors could find no good evidence to support the link, but also no evidence to firmly refute it. This doesn't always mean there is no evidence. In most cases, there is some report linking the events from the adverse-event reporting system. But when the authors looked into it, it seemed unlikely that the two were related.

This is a somewhat frustrating conclusion. Basically, whatever you thought before (in statistics speak, your "prior beliefs") is what you'll think after seeing the evidence. If people come in thinking vaccines are safe, then there is nothing here to argue against that. Conversely, if they come in thinking vaccines are unsafe, there is nothing here to help refute that. For people who really want to believe that vaccines are damaging, this nonevidence may be seen to support their beliefs—as in, "We cannot rule out a link between MMR and multiple sclerosis." Based on this standard, you cannot rule out a link between fingernail cutting and multiple sclerosis. The only difference is that no one believes the latter link exists in the first place.

In general, it is very difficult to *prove* there is no relationship between two events. If we are worried about a very small relationship, we'd need huge sample sizes to statistically reject it. We don't often have these. It would be great to have more evidence, but the IOM can only work with what they have.

Of the seventeen cases where the IOM thought they could draw conclusions, fourteen were judged to either convincingly support a relationship or favor acceptance. This may seem scary, but it is important to look carefully at what the risks are.

First, for many of the vaccines (all but the DTaP vaccines), there is a risk of allergic reaction. This is extremely rare (about 0.22 in 100,000 vaccines) and can be treated with Benadryl or, in an extreme case, an EpiPen. Allergic reactions account for half the documented risks in the report.

Second, fainting sometimes occurs after vaccination, mostly among adolescents. It is unclear what the mechanism is, but fainting does not have long-term consequences. This accounts for another two of the convincingly supported risks.

There are then several cases in which vaccines are linked to more serious risks. However, in these cases, the risks are generally *extremely tiny*. An example is the link between the MMR vaccine and "measles inclusions body encephalitis." This condition is a very serious long-term complication of measles infection that occurs in people who are immune-compromised. It is very rare, nearly always fatal, and is a well-known complication of actual measles infection. The question for the IOM report was whether someone could also get this after measles vaccination. In the report, the authors examine three cases in which subsequent testing of children diagnosed with this disease showed that they were very likely exposed to measles through vaccination, not through an actual case of measles.

Given this evidence—that we know this to be a risk of the measles virus, and that the children in these three cases weren't exposed to actual measles—the report concluded that in these cases, it is likely the vaccine caused the disease.

This relationship is categorized as "convincingly supports." It is very important to be clear, though, that this doesn't mean this is a risk everyone should be concerned about. It arises only for children who are immune-compromised, and even then it is vanishingly rare. There are just *three* case reports in the history of vaccination. If your child has an immune issue, you'll know, and you'll talk through vaccination with your doctor. For healthy children, this simply isn't a risk you should consider in your vaccine calculus.

Similar issues arise for immune-compromised children who get the chicken pox vaccine. Again, these complications are extremely rare. There is a vaccine link here, but this is far from saying these are scenarios you should be actively worried about it. They are not.

There is, finally, one vaccine risk that is more common and, while not serious, can be scary. Specifically, the MMR vaccine is linked with febrile seizures—seizures that occur in infants or young children in association with a high fever. They typically do not have long-term consequences, but are very scary in the moment.

These are common enough that we can study their relationships to vaccines using large datasets of children. About 2 to 3 percent of children in the US will have a febrile seizure before they are five years old (most of these are not vaccine associated).[7] A number of studies find that these seizures are about twice as likely in the period ten days or so after the MMR vaccine.[8] They are actually more likely for children who get their first MMR dose later (i.e., older than one year); this is a reason to vaccinate on time, rather than to delay.

One thing the IOM report does not cover is infant crankiness, which, as your doctor will probably tell you, is a result of vaccines for many babies. I learned about this link the hard way. We inexplicably scheduled a large student brunch at our house for a few hours after Penelope's first vaccinations. We also failed to have any infant Tylenol stocked. Jesse ended up serving pastries to the students in our dining room on his own, while I wrestled a hysterically screaming baby into the Baby Bjorn for a walk to CVS. Not our finest afternoon. Still, by the next morning, the storm had passed.

This crankiness—often accompanied by a fever—may be annoying, but it is not something to worry about. Your baby is working to create antibodies to a virus, and this work has some side effects. But not ones to be concerned about. Just make sure you have infant Tylenol around.

This covers the data-supported risks of vaccines. What about the relationships that are *not* supported in the data? The IOM report explicitly rejects several links. One of them is the link between the MMR vaccine and autism, the link suggested by Andrew Wakefield in his *Lancet* paper.

There are a number of big studies of this relationship. The largest of them includes 537,000 children—all the children born in Denmark from 1991 to 1998. In the Danish data, the authors were able to link vaccination information to later diagnosis of autism or autism-spectrum disorders. They found no evidence that vaccinated children are more likely to be autistic; if anything, the results suggest vaccinated children are *less* likely to be diagnosed with autism.[9]

There are many similar studies; some are included in the IOM report, others postdate it. One study focuses on children who have an older sibling with autism and who are therefore more likely to have it themselves. Again, researchers found no link with the MMR vaccine.[10]

There is no mechanism by which this would occur, and controlled studies in monkeys also show no plausible relationship.[11] *At the end of the day, there is simply no reason to think autism and vaccinations are linked.*[12]

It is not fair to say there are no risks associated with vaccination at all. Your child may well get a fever. It is also possible (although really quite unlikely) that this fever would lead to a seizure. It is also possible (although, again, very, very unlikely) that they could have an allergic reaction.

But it is reasonable to say there is no evidence of significant long-term consequences of vaccines for healthy children.

VACCINE EFFICACY

Those of us in the US are lucky to live in a place where most people do get vaccinated, and cases of vaccine-preventable disease are rare. Few children get measles or mumps, and a few more get pertussis, but not many. If people stopped vaccinating, this would not be true anymore. All these diseases exist around us, and in the absence of vaccination, infection would be common.

Vaccination does a very good job of protecting against disease, but it is not perfect. For pertussis, for example, immunity wears off over time. Despite this, studies consistently show that even in places with a high overall vaccination rate, children who are vaccinated are less likely to become infected than those who are not.[13] During a 2015 measles outbreak that originated in Disneyland, the affected children were largely those whose parents had not had them vaccinated.

If you are nervous about vaccines, despite the evidence above, there may be a temptation to rely on the actions of others to prevent your own child's illness. This is the idea of "herd immunity": if a large enough share of people are vaccinated, then a disease cannot get a foothold, and the whole population—the herd—is immune. And it is true that if your child is literally the *only* child who is not vaccinated in your area, and you never travel anywhere that there are other unvaccinated children, your child is pretty much guaranteed not to get these diseases.

But how feasible is that? For one thing, many areas of the US have vaccination rates that are below the rate needed for herd immunity: in some pockets, MMR vaccine rates are around 80 percent; you need a vaccination rate of at least 90 percent to have a hope of herd immunity. Pertussis is even more common and requires even higher vaccination rates to deliver herd immunity. As a result, about half the counties in the US have at least one pertussis case every year. Many have more. Even if you focus only on the risks to your child in particular, there are good reasons to vaccinate.

And it is worth saying that vaccination is pro-social. If everyone tried to do what economists call "free-ride" and not vaccinate their children, then we'd have no vaccination and a lot of disease. Some children cannot be vaccinated due to immune deficiencies, cancer, or other complications; healthy children getting vaccinated protects these vulnerable kids.

Most of us born in the past forty years have not known a time when the diseases for which we vaccinate our children were common. Maybe you've heard of one or two children getting measles, but they probably got better, since the vast majority of people recover from the disease. Most of us do not know anyone who died from a vaccine-preventable disease. But it can happen, and when these diseases are common, it does.

And it is worth remembering that people can have terrible reactions even to diseases that are mostly not that serious. We probably remember chicken pox as a pretty benign, if itchy, illness. But prior to the development of a vaccine, it caused about a hundred deaths and nine thousand hospitalizations a year. Pertussis deaths—ten to twenty a year—occur even now, mostly among babies who are too young to be vaccinated yet, and are therefore relying on other people's vaccination behavior to protect them.

Particularly when you haven't seen or experienced widespread illness, vaccines can seem like a waste of time—like you're sticking needles into your kid for no reason. But the fact of the matter is, they are not. Vaccines prevent disease, suffering, and death.

DELAYED VACCINATION SCHEDULES

Some vaccine-anxious parents favor a delayed vaccine schedule, in which children receive vaccines spaced out over a longer period of time rather than being given several at once.

There is no reason to do this, given the evidence on vaccine safety that I outlined earlier, and in fact, the risk of a febrile seizure actually increases if the MMR vaccine is given later.[14] Delaying vaccines will not help to avoid any of the limited adverse events attributed to vaccination. It also takes more of your time to visit the doctor repeatedly for shots, and your kid will not like them.

The only value I can see in a delayed vaccination schedule is that it may encourage some parents to vaccinate when they wouldn't otherwise. Later is better than never, although in many cases—the rotavirus vaccines, for example—there are good reasons to start on time. The first hepatitis B vaccines are given in the first couple of days of a child's life and, in the unlikely case of undiagnosed hepatitis B in the mother, can prevent long-term development of liver cancer in the child.[15] So there are reasons to start on time.

Some doctors also worry that offering delayed vaccinations gives the impression that people should be nervous about vaccines, that there *is* something to worry about. Could that encourage fewer people to vaccinate? It is an interesting theory, but there is not much evidence to support it.

From an individual parent standpoint, the bottom line is that there is simply no reason for delay.

The Bottom Line

- Vaccinations are safe.
  - A very small share of people have allergic reactions, which are treatable.
  - There are some extremely rare adverse events, most of which occur in immune-compromised children.
  - The only more common risks are fever and febrile seizures, which are also rare and do not do long-term harm.
  - There is no evidence of a link between vaccines and autism, and much evidence to refute such a link.
- Vaccines prevent children from getting sick.

9

Stay-at-Home Mom?
Stay-at-Work Mom?

Nothing in the Mommy Wars takes on as much weight as the choice to return to work or not. The title of this chapter comes from a friend whose son was once asked at school, "What kind of mom do you have? I have a stay-at-home mom," to which my friend's son responded, "Oh, I have a stay-at-work mom."

The phrasing of this—what *kind* of mom do you have?—encapsulates much of the tension. Many of us have the feeling that the choice of what we do during the day is going to determine, at a deep level, what kind of mom (and person) we are.

Additionally, or perhaps as a result, this is an area with a tremendous amount of associated tension and unhappiness. Women who work (some of them, anyway) tell me they feel guilty about not being with their child every minute. Those who do not work (some of them, anyway) tell me they feel isolated and resentful at times. And even when we are happy with our choices at a personal level, it can feel as though there's a lot of judgment coming from both directions:

"Why aren't you available to go on the school field trip? Oh, I see, you'll be at work. It's too bad—Petunia was asking about you."

"So what do you do? Oh, you're *just* home with the kids? I could never do that—I'd let so many people down at work."

People, this has got to stop. All cross-parental judgment is unhelpful and counterproductive, and this is no different.

For one thing, the whole premise of the discussion is gendered in an unhelpful way. The choice of whether to have a parent stay home is one your family will need to make. But why does it have to be Mom? It doesn't. Framing this through the stay-at-home-mom lens makes it harder for people to think "stay-at-home dad" is a valid choice. But it should be. Never mind that sometimes a family has two moms. Or two dads. Or only one parent.

So let's start by just framing this not as "What kind of mom will you be?" but "What is the optimal configuration of adult work hours for your household?" Less catchy, yes, but also perhaps more helpful for decision-making.

Second, this discussion ignores the fact that this really isn't a choice for some families. There are plenty of people in the US who cannot get by— and by "get by" I mean have a place to live and put food on the table— without all the adults in the household working.

If your family is lucky enough to have a choice, the goal of this chapter is to try to give you a way to think about it. Ideally, this starts with decision theory and hard data, not with guilt and shame.

STRUCTURING THE DECISION

How should you think about the choice of working? I'd argue it has three components.

1. What is best for your child? (Let's take "best" to mean likely to help promote their long-term life success, happiness, etc.)
2. What do you want to do?
3. What are the implications of your choice for the family budget?

People often talk about 1 and 3, and I'll spend some time on those in this chapter. But I'd like to encourage you to also think about 2. That is, you should think about whether you *want* to work. It is common for people to say they work "because I have to" or stay home "because I have to." And in either case, that can sometimes be true. But I think it is not true as much as people say it.

And this is a problem. It should be okay to say you made this choice because you wanted to work or wanted to stay home.

I'll say it: I am lucky enough to not *have to* work, in the sense that Jesse and I could change how we organize our life to live on one income. I work because I like to. I love my kids! They are amazing. But I wouldn't be happy staying home with them. I've figured out that my happiness-maximizing allocation is something like eight hours of work and three hours of kids a day.

It isn't that I like my job more than my kids overall—if I had to pick, the kids would win every time. But the "marginal value" of time with my kids declines fast. In part, this is because kids are exhausting. The first hour with them is amazing, the second less good, and by hour four I'm ready for a glass of wine or, even better, some time with my research.

My job doesn't have this feature. Yes, the eighth hour is less fun than the seventh, but the highs are not as high and the lows are not as low. The physical and emotional challenges of work pale in comparison to the physical and emotional challenges of being an on-scene parent. The eighth hour at my job is better than the fifth hour with the kids on a typical day. And that is why I have a job. Because I like it.

It should be okay to say this. Just like it should be okay to say that you stay home with your kids because that is what you want to do. I'm well aware that many people don't want to be an economist for eight hours a day. We shouldn't have to say we're staying home for children's optimal development, or at least, that shouldn't be the only factor in the decision. "This is the lifestyle I prefer" or "This is what works for my family" are both okay reasons to make choices! So before you even get into reading what the evidence says is "best" for your child or thinking about the family budget, you—and your partner, or any other caregiving adults in the house—should think about what you would really *like* to do.

And then you can think about the data and the constraints.

I'm going to start by talking about the choice to work at all—first, its impacts on your child, and second, a bit about how to think about its impacts on your budget. At the end of the chapter, I'll spend some time on the question of early parental leave and whether there is any guidance about how much leave to take if you do plan to return to work.

IMPACTS OF PARENTAL EMPLOYMENT ON CHILD OUTCOMES

Let's start with the first question: Is it better (or worse) for your child's development to have one parent stay home?

This is an extremely difficult question to answer. Why? First, households that choose to have a parent stay home are different from those that do not. And these differences, totally independent of a parent staying home or not, are likely to influence what happens to the children in those households.

Second, what your child does while you are at work is likely to matter tremendously. Once they are older, they'll all go to school, but if we are talking about young kids, the outcomes will be influenced by whether they are in a good care environment (the next chapter will spend some time on how to think about childcare if you do choose to return to work).

Finally, working generally means money. And money also may be good for your family, or open up opportunities you and your children wouldn't have otherwise. So it is a challenge to separate the impact of income from the impact of parental time.

Even with these caveats, we can dive into the data.

We can start with a place where we do have some causal evidence: the impact of a parent staying home in the first couple of years. I'll talk below about maternity leave specifically, and the question of, say, no maternity leave versus six weeks or three months of leave. But there is also a set of literature that estimates whether it matters for kids if parents are home for, say, a year versus six months, or fifteen months versus a year. This comes from Europe and Canada, where policies have been introduced at various times to extend maternity leave into these ranges. (Let's leave aside our anger that the US makes people fight for six weeks while these other places are arguing about one year versus two.)

In this literature, the authors are exploiting a change in a *policy*, not differences in choices, so they can be more confident about their conclusions. Extending maternity leave from six months to a year makes some women stay home for a year when they would otherwise have stayed home for six months. By comparing the outcomes of children who are born in the "six month" maternity leave policy to those born in the "year" policy, we can learn about the effects of maternity leave without worrying about underlying differences across parents.

The bottom line from this literature is that these parental-leave extensions have no effect on child outcomes.[1] No effects on children's test scores in school, on income later in life, or on anything else. In many cases, these studies have very long follow-up periods. We can say, for example, that one year of parental leave versus two years doesn't influence a child's high school test scores or earnings in early adulthood.

This evidence focuses on parents working in the first years. If we want to see the impact of parents working when their children are older, we are limited to studies that estimate correlations, not causal impacts. Some studies do exist, though, and when we look for evidence on schooling—test scores, school completion—these correlations tend to be about zero.[2] Two parents working full time has a similar effect to one parent working and one not.

There is sometimes a bit of nuance in the results. One thing that is commonly seen is that children in families where one parent works part time and the other works full time tend to perform best in school—better than children whose parents both work full time or who have one parent who doesn't work at all.[3] This could be due to the working configuration, but I think it's more likely due to differences between these families.[4]

Second, studies tend to find that the impacts of both parents working are positive (i.e., working is better) for kids from poorer families, and less positive (or even slightly negative) for children from richer families.[5] The outcomes here are things like test scores, school achievement, and even obesity.

Researchers tend to interpret this as saying that in poor households, the income from working is important for child outcomes. Whereas in richer households, the lost time doing "enriching" things with a parent is more important. This is possible, although since these estimates are still just correlations, it is challenging to read so much into the data. And even if we do admit this interpretation, it highlights the importance of the child's activities, not the parent leave configuration.

A final note is that some people have argued that if both parents work—and, specifically, if Mom works—their daughters are more likely to work in the long run and show less evidence of sex stereotypes.[6] These are interesting ideas, and certainly it might be nice to think your kids are modeling themselves after you. But most of this data comes from comparing the US to Europe, so it is hard to know if the effects are attributable to maternal employment or other differences.

Tying this all together, my view is that the weight of the evidence suggests the net effects of working on child development are small or zero. Depending on your household configuration, these effects could be a little positive or a little negative. But this isn't the decision that is going to make or break your child's future success (if there is any decision that would at all).

PARENTAL LEAVE

The United States has subpar maternity leave policies. Many European countries give months—even a year or two—of paid, or partially paid, leave with guaranteed job security. Many people in the US have no paid leave at all, and even unpaid leave (say, through the Family Medical Leave Act, or FMLA) is typically capped at twelve weeks and is available to only about 60 percent of working people.

This has slowly started to change. Some states—notably California, New York, Rhode Island (shout-out!), New Jersey, Washington, and Washington, DC—have introduced paid-leave provisions. These benefits typically extend only six to twelve weeks, but they're at least something. And there are discussions of paid leave at the federal level, although nothing has yet come of them.

If you are lucky, your job provides some paid leave. This could be up to three or four months, depending on where you work, or may be less. Technology firms have been working to set an example by providing up to four months of paid leave for women *and* men. Of course, you might not work at Facebook.

Parental leave appears to be beneficial. There is a growing body of evidence suggesting that babies do better when their mothers take some maternity leave. In the US, for example, research has shown that when the FMLA was introduced, babies did better. Premature birth went down, as did infant mortality.[7] The mechanism may be that if moms are off work with small babies, they are better able to get care for them when they are sick. This policy may also have encouraged leave before birth for women with difficult pregnancies, which could account for the effect on premature birth.

Other work on this shows similar results. When researchers look at everything together, they generally conclude that early maternity leave is beneficial.[8]

These benefits seem to focus on infancy, not later in life.[9] However, one study that looked at kids in Norway showed that introducing a four-month paid maternity leave for moms led to higher education and even higher wages for their children when they grew up. These long-term effects were largest for the children of moms who were less well-off financially.[10]

This is all to say that if your job offers parental leave, you should take it. If it does not, it is worth considering whether you can take some unpaid leave. The FMLA gives you the right to twelve weeks of unpaid leave, assuming you've worked a sufficient amount during the previous year and your firm employs at least fifty people. Although the leave is unpaid, your employer must keep you on insurance coverage and hold your job (or a comparable one) for you until you return.

Although unpaid leave can be challenging for many families, and there are no federal maternity leave benefits in the US, it is worth exploring whether your state offers benefits. As noted above, a bunch of states do have paid-leave provisions, and hopefully more will introduce them over time. You can sometimes put together multiple state programs—temporary disability insurance plus paid family leave, for example—to create a longer paid period. Even if you can cobble together only a few weeks, the benefits for your child may be worth it.

BUDGETING

The final consideration in parental work is the impact on your family budget. This issue is complicated. It requires thinking about the income of each parent, and the cost of childcare. And ideally you'd think about both of these in both the short and long term.

Childcare is expensive, and most of it is paid in "after-tax" income. This means that your income needs to be considerably more than the cost of childcare to break even.

To see how this works, think about a family whose total income is $100,000, with each parent making $50,000. This family brings home about $85,000 after taxes.[11] If both parents work and the family pays $1,500 a month for childcare, their total disposable income after childcare is taken into account is $67,000 a year. If one parent stays home, the family makes less (about $46,000 in take-home pay), but does not pay for childcare. The difference in take-home income is about half what it would be if the couple did not have any children.

This calculus becomes more complicated if childcare is more expensive. A full-time nanny, especially if you pay the legally required taxes and live in an expensive area, can run to $40,000 or $50,000 a year. For my example family above, that would completely wipe out one parent's income. They'd be better off financially with one parent staying home.

This can also be true if one parent makes more than the other. In our example family, let's imagine that the total income is the same, but now one parent is making $70,000 and the other $30,000. The parent making $30,000 is bringing home $25,500 a year; after the childcare expenses, the difference in disposable income with that parent working versus not is just $7,500.

These are just examples—your personal financial situation may be quite different. But a first step in figuring this out is to actually confront the situation. What would your family income be with one parent staying home versus both working? What are the realistic childcare costs? To do this well you probably want to use an online tax calculator (or a tax preparer) to help you think about the impact on your taxes of childcare cost deductions and so on.

This is the first piece of the calculation. But it shouldn't be the last. There are at least two more things to think about.

First, the calculus changes as your child ages. Your kids will get less expensive as they grow up. School-age kids tend to cost less—public schools are free, for example. And if you stay in the workforce, your income will probably go up (this depends a bit on your job, but is true for many people). This means that even if working doesn't seem like a good deal for the first few years, it may be a good deal in the long run. Of course, you could stop working when the kids are little and then return to work later—many people do—but this is easier to do in some jobs than others. And there is no guarantee that you won't take a substantial salary hit when you do come back—to say nothing of the lost retirement savings.

There is no blanket rule for how to think of the short- and long-run trade-offs; it is simply to say that you shouldn't limit your budget thinking to the ages of zero to three.

Second, you want to think about what economists call the "marginal value of money." Let's say your family would be better off in terms of income if you worked. You can calculate this in a dollar value, but that doesn't necessarily tell you how much happier you'd be. You really want to think about how much your family would value that money in terms of what economists call "utility," aka happiness. How different will your life be? What will you buy with this money? If it doesn't make you happier, then it isn't worth much, even if it is money.

MAKING A CHOICE

Whether to have all adults in the household work outside the home is not an easy choice for most people, and it is nearly impossible to give blanket advice. The data suggests that—putting aside early maternity leave, which has some significant benefits—there is not much evidence that having a stay-at-home parent positively or negatively affects child development.

This means it really comes down to what works for your family. This includes thinking about your budget, but also thinking about what you want. Does one parent want to be home with the kid or not? In a sense, this is probably the main consideration, but it is also the most complex and hard to predict. Before you have a child, it's pretty difficult to tell if you'll want to be with them all the time.

Some people love being with their baby every minute and cannot imagine being away.

Some people eagerly look forward to returning to work on Monday morning, even if they love their kids just as much.

And this may change as the children age. Some people really love babies. I have found that as my kids get older, I enjoy being with them more. I still do not want to be a stay-at-home parent, but I think I'd like it more now than I would have when they were younger. Try to be honest with yourself about what you want.

None of this is very helpful to you in making a choice. Sorry! Ultimately, you are on your own.

To conclude: By acknowledging that the choice to stay home or not is just that—a choice, with factors pushing you in various directions—we can perhaps start to move away from the judgmental attitude that seems to crop up on both sides of the aisle. I'd like to be able to say that I choose to have a job because that is what I want, and I'd like friends to be able to say they choose to stay home because that is what they want. And I'd like us to be able to say both these things without my being tempted to look down my nose at those friends and their being tempted to imply that my children will not have the best start in life.

Is that so much to ask? I think it is not.

The Bottom Line

- Babies benefit from their mothers taking some maternity leave. However, there is little evidence suggesting that having a stay-at-home parent after the parental leave period has either good or bad consequences for children.
- Decisions about whether to have a parent stay home should consider your preferences, along with consequences for your family budget in both the short and long term.
- Stop judging people!

Who Should Take Care
of the Baby?

I f you do decide to, as I said previously, "have all the adults in the household work outside the home," you are then immediately faced with the next question: What on earth will you do with your baby?

When I was newly pregnant with Penelope, Jesse and I took a trip to give some seminars in Sweden. Between bouts of vomiting in our entirely IKEA-outfitted apartment (did you know IKEA makes shampoo?), I could not help but notice with envy the childcare setup that seemed to be available to Swedish parents.

Parents in Sweden get a lot of parental leave, but in addition, once they go back to work, there are a variety of excellent government-provided childcare options. As we walked around Stockholm, there were many groups of small children trekking between parks, hanging on to ropes to stay together. It looked awesome! If the Swedes had offered us a job, I probably would have argued for decamping there, at least until Penelope was ready for school. They did not.

Back in the US, childcare is not as simple. There are many options, but no default government-provided option as there is in many European countries. This is the case for many reasons, but it's probably best understood as politics. These European countries provide more services of all kinds—health care, for example—and childcare is a part of that. This is also a case where countries are probably drawn to doing what they have long done. People in Sweden expect good government-provided childcare. People in the US might wish for it, but they don't expect it.

If you don't live somewhere with an obvious childcare option, you've got to figure this out for yourself. Day care or a nanny are the most standard setups, but you could have a family member pitch in, or have some hybrid of these. Even within these basic options, there are many variations. Take day care. What kind is right for you? Home day care? Center-based day care? If you hire a nanny, what kind of nanny? When looking for our first nanny, a reference described one candidate as "not a flash-card nanny." I didn't know that was a kind. Did I want that kind?

I'm going to argue that you can simplify this whole thing, though, by taking a page from the decision-theory playbook. More specifically, you need a decision tree. Here's an example—a kind of parenting decision tree. For the purposes of this chapter, we'll focus on outside childcare options. If you have an extended family member who can help, you can add another limb to your tree.

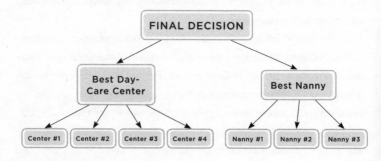

In economics, we teach people to "solve the tree." To do this, you work backward from the bottom. First, decide what nanny you would want if you *had* to have a nanny (in this case, I gave you three choices). Then you've solved that leaf of the tree. Then decide what kind of day care you would want if you *had* to have day care (here, you've got four choices). Then compare those two.

Now, rather than comparing the wide range of options in each category, you are facing a very specific choice: Do I prefer my "optimal" day-care setup or my "optimal" nanny setup?

So there is your theory. Of course, theory doesn't tell us the right answer, only how to think about the problem. To get to the answer, we need to combine theory with evidence—specifically, evidence on different childcare options, and how to compare them.

THE DAY-CARE OPTION

Imagine we find ourselves in the left-hand side of the tree: day care. How do you choose the best one?

Data to help with this comes from studies like the National Institute of Child Health and Human Development Study of Early Child Care and Youth Development (I will call this the NICHD study going forward, just to save some words).

The NICHD is a longitudinal study (meaning it follows kids over time) of more than one thousand children, designed to evaluate the impacts of various types of childcare (day care, nanny, family member) on child development. NICHD researchers were interested in outcomes like language development and behavior problems. This study will be useful in comparing day care to nanny as well, but for the moment we can focus on the comparison across day care options.

In the study, researchers actually went into the day-care centers where the study children were enrolled and evaluated them. They sat in the classroom and observed the teachers and recorded other facts about the day care. And then they ranked them, determining which day cares were higher "quality" than others.

They were looking for very specific qualities in a high-quality day care, which we'll discuss in a moment. But before getting into that, it's useful to see how quality matters.

A first paper using this data looks at the relationship between child-care and cognitive ability and behavior issues at the age of four.[1] To do this, the authors effectively compared children who went to higher-quality day cares to those who went to lower-quality day cares. Day-care attendance is through childhood up to the age of four (they may still be in the evaluated day care, or may have moved on).

The authors found that attending higher-quality day care strongly correlated with better child language development: kids who went to better day cares seem to talk more. When they looked at behavior problems, though, there did not seem to be a relationship to day-care quality in either direction—the effect was about zero.

The researchers doing this study followed the children through sixth grade and continued to find that day-care quality is associated with better vocabulary outcomes, but not with behavior.[2]

It should be clear by this point in the book that there is an obvious issue with this analysis, which is that day-care quality also relates to other features of the family. On average, higher-quality day care is more expensive, and therefore, a different set of kids are enrolled—kids who, for example, come from better-off families. It is therefore hard to know which outcomes to attribute to the family and which to the day care.

An advantage of this particular study is the ability to control extensively for family background. They did home visits, so they could evaluate something about the quality of parenting as well. Parenting matters a lot—way more than day care—but their day-care results remained even after adjusting for the parenting differences they observed. Of course, concerns remain about the possible role of parental characteristics we do not observe.

With these caveats in mind, the evidence reinforces the commonsense intuition that if you are going to send your child to day care, it should be a good one. Leading to the obvious question: How do you know if it's good? One way to get a sense of this is to go back to the NICHD study and consider how the researchers evaluated quality. You may not be able to replicate their methods exactly, but you can at least get a sense of what they were looking for.

Let's start with what they were not looking for: what I call "fancy" day-care features. There is no box to tick for "early Mandarin exposure" or "organic snacks." They also did not focus on things like whether the day care tried to teach kids facts about penguins. Overwhelmingly, the evaluation of day-care quality focused on the interactions between the providers and the children.

The quality evaluation has several parts. First, there is effectively a checklist of questions on safety, fun, and "individualization." Here's a simple version:

Safety	Fun	Individualization
▪ No exposed outlets, cords, fans, etc.	▪ Toys can be reached by kids	▪ Kid has own crib
▪ Safe cribs	▪ Floor space available for crawlers to play	▪ Each infant is assigned to one of the teachers
▪ Written emergency plan	▪ 3 different types of "large-muscle materials" available (balls, rocking horse)	▪ Child development is assessed formally at least every 6 months
▪ Disposable towels available	▪ 3 types of music materials available	▪ Infants offered toys appropriate for their development level
▪ Eating area away from diaper area	▪ "Special activities" (i.e., water play, sponge painting)	▪ Teachers have at least 1 hour a week for team planning
▪ Toys washed each day	▪ 3 materials for outdoor infant play	
▪ Teacher knows about infant illnesses		

Most of these things can be easily observed and recorded on a day-care tour, and the checklist is basically the same for center-based or home-based day care.

In addition, they also assessed quality by watching the child at day care several times. The observation periods are fairly short—a burst of four ten-minute observation periods over the course of a half day. This is probably harder to replicate, but if you are considering a day care, it would not be unreasonable to ask if you can quietly observe from the sidelines for ten to fifteen minutes. I would probably avoid actually bringing a numerical observation sheet, but, you know, that's up to you.

What were the observers looking for? First, some basic things. Is the adult (or adults) available and interacting with the children (i.e., are they on their phone, or are they down on the floor with the babies)? Do they have positive physical contact with the children (reinforcing good behavior with a hug, holding the baby)?

Then there are some questions on developmental stimulation. Does the adult read to the children? Do they talk to them? Do they respond when the baby makes a noise? ("Gah!" "That's right, that's a hippo. Hip-po. Do you want to hold the hippo? Here you go!")

Third, there is behavior. All babies and children act out at various times. The question is, how does the adult respond? Do they respond to negative behavior by physically restraining the child or children involved (the researchers' question specifically is, do they "restrict them in a physical container")? Do they hit? Do they speak negatively to the child? These would all be (very) bad signs.

Finally, there is a set of observations about what the children are doing. Do they seem physically well (not hungry, not wearing a poopy diaper, etc.)? Are they getting some time interacting with adults? Are they, heaven forbid, watching TV?

At the end of the observation, the observer is also supposed to record some general feelings. Is the day care child-centered? That is, do the adults seem like they are really focused on what the kids want to do, listening to them and responding to them? Or are the adults just going through the motions, mostly focused on each other and not on the kids? Do the children and adults seem to have a positive and loving relationship? Do the children seem well-adjusted and happy, or do they seem afraid and cringe at the sight of the adult?

You are (presumably) not a trained day-care observer. On the other hand, many of these characteristics are things you could look for on your own. It is very unlikely a caregiver would hit a child in front of you, but negative affect and a lack of warmth aren't actually very hard to pick up on. And it's hard to fake the opposite.

A reasonable question to ask is whether this is all just a way to say you should pick the most expensive day care you can afford. It is true that quality and price are correlated: more expensive day cares are going to be, on average, higher quality. But the main component of quality—how the care providers interact with the children—is not about price.

THE NANNY OPTION

Okay, so we've solved the day-care node (or at least done our best). We've done our clipboard evaluations and found the best possible day-care option.

Now, what about the nanny?

The NICHD study evaluates the quality of at-home (i.e., nanny or other non-mom family member) childcare, with the same results: higher-quality childcare, as determined by the metrics they can measure, is better. However, quality in this case is even harder to evaluate than for day care.

The study uses a similar evaluation period and checklist to see if the caregiver is responsive to the child, if there are toys and books around, if there is yelling or hitting (both bad). Unfortunately, it is likely to be much harder to do a reliable evaluation of a single adult–child interaction, where it will be obvious the researcher is there, watching the caregiver, than at a day care, where you can more easily fade into the background.

In addition, even more so than in the case of day care, the quality ratings are likely to be related to socioeconomic status in a way that overstates the importance of caregiver quality. One of the questions—for example—is whether the child has at least three books. But this is a feature of the family, not the nanny.

Beyond this, there is simply very little concrete guidance about how to find and evaluate a nanny. Perhaps the most useful piece of advice I got in doing this was to talk to references (of course) and try to evaluate not only whether they liked the person but also whether the person doing the referring seemed like me. Were we people with similar needs?

It can also be useful to have candidates answer some basic questions in writing. When you're interviewing someone, it can be hard to remember everything you wanted to ask. If you use an agency, they'll often provide a suggested questionnaire. If not, you can find some online.

Hiring a nanny is a bit of a leap of faith, and you may have to trust your gut. When my daughter was three, we moved, pretty abruptly, from Chicago to Providence. We left our beloved nanny, Madu, in Chicago, and had to look for someone else on a tight time frame. We ended up hiring Becky without ever having met her in person, after just two phone calls and having her meet my brother. It just felt right—which it was—although this is hard to square with my ever-eager desire for data.

DAY CARE VS. NANNY

At this stage of the decision tree, you should have chosen your optimal day care and nanny structure. Now to compare them. Is one necessarily better?

One problem with the data is that many studies that look at day care, in particular, implicitly or explicitly compare it to the option of being home with Mom. This is an interesting comparison—see the previous chapter—but it isn't exactly the same as comparing day care with a nanny.

The NICHD study is our best option here. This study *does* explicitly compare nanny-type arrangements to "center-based childcare," and makes an attempt, although it is, of course, imperfect, to adjust for differences in family background.

The paper that summarizes the effects on children through age four and a half looks at cognitive and language development, and at behavior problems.[3] On the cognitive side, the results are mixed. More months in day care before eighteen months are associated with slightly lower cognitive scores by four and a half years old, but more time in care after that is associated with *higher* cognitive outcomes.

It is hard to know why this is. It could be that very early on the one-on-one attention enhances early language development, but at older ages, children in day care are likely to spend more time on skills like letters, numbers, and social integration than children cared for by nannies or stay-at-home parents. But this is speculation. It is also possible that these are just correlations—that they are not causal at all.

Studies that combine this suggest that, overall, the effect is positive—that kids who are in day care for more time over this entire period have better language and cognitive outcomes at four and a half.[4]

On the behavior side, there are small associations between behavior problems and more time in day care at all ages, although the authors caution that these effects are fairly minimal and all the children were in the "normal" behavior range.

These effects—both the (slightly) positive cognitive effects and the (slightly) negative behavior effects—seem to persist through the early grades at school, although they fade substantially by third or fifth grade.[5]

This is only one study, but the effects are mimicked in other contexts. Day care is associated with better cognitive outcomes[6] and slightly worse behavior.[7] The cognitive-outcome effects seem to be concentrated in care that occurs at slightly older ages. There is a variety of evidence for this last point—for example, the evidence for the effectiveness of the federal Head Start program is based on studies showing that preschool hours enhance school readiness.

There are various other things evaluated in these studies. One is "infant attachment." Are kids in day care less attached to their moms? No, they are not. Quality of parenting matters for this, but day-care time makes no difference.[8]

A final data-driven comparison is with illness. Kids who are in day care are more likely to get sick.[9] These are not serious illnesses, more like

colds and fevers, stomach flu, and so on. On the plus side, these early ex-
posures seem to confer some immunity, with children who were in day
care for more years as toddlers having *fewer* colds in early elementary
school.[10]

In all this we come back again and again to two things: First, parenting matters. Much more consistent than any of the associations in these
studies is the association between parenting and child outcomes. Having
books in your house and reading them to your kid is going to matter much
more than what books they have at day care. This seems to be true even
though your child probably spends as many waking hours with their care
providers as with you. I don't think we know precisely why this is the case,
although it may be that you as the parent are the most consistent influence
your child has. Second, childcare quality matters much more than which
type of childcare you have. A high-quality day care is likely to be better
than a low-quality nanny, and vice versa.

The choice of childcare arrangement is also not *just* about your child.
Ultimately, you have to figure out what works for your family. This intro-
duces considerations beyond the cognitive development ones.

First, there is cost. On average, a nanny is more expensive than day
care (although this may not always be true). An arrangement where you
share a nanny with another family may be a way to offset some of the
nanny costs. This is a question for your budget.

What is the right share of your budget to spend on childcare? There is
no one answer. The way we thought about it—this is really getting into the
weeds of economist parenting, a place where no one may want to be—is
back to the "marginal utility of money." Let's say that the difference between a nanny share and having your own nanny is $10,000 a year for 3
years, so $30,000 total. Obviously, if you prefer the nanny share, it's an
easy choice.

But if you prefer not to share the nanny, you want to think about how
much that money is worth to you. The key is to think about its marginal
value. Yes, this is a lot of money (childcare is SO EXPENSIVE). But that's
not the relevant question. The question is what would you do if you had

that money? What is the next best, non-childcare, use of these funds? This is the same question I encouraged you to ask about having a parent stay home.

It may be that the difference is in how nice a house or apartment you have. It may mean a difference in some vacation choices. It may mean less savings—you're then trading your retirement plans for something now. There isn't an easy choice. But by being explicit about what else you'd do with the money, you can at least frame the decision a bit more concretely: Would you rather have your own nanny, or two vacations a year, or more retirement savings?

Beyond budget, there is the question of convenience. Is there a day care close by (either to home or work), or will you have to drive far out of your way for drop-off? And what are your options if your child gets sick? At home, care can still work with a sick kid (also, kids get sick less at home), but day care cannot. What are your backup options?

One of the best pieces of parenting advice I got from my friend Nancy was this: Regardless of what childcare you choose, have a plan for who is in charge when the nanny or the kid is sick. Fighting about who will miss work in the moment is a bad idea.

Finally, you might simply feel more comfortable with one of these options or the other. That is a good reason to choose that option! Many people express discomfort at the idea of one person being with their child, in their house, all day. Your relationship with an in-home caregiver can be complex. If you have a nanny, one day your child will call you by their name. Will this make you feel bad? There is no uniform answer to this, but it is something to think about in advance.

This is a family decision. If all the adults in the household choose to work outside the home, you need to be happy with your childcare. You'll spend enough time thinking about your children while you're at work anyway, and if you are worried about them all day, you won't get anything done. Finding an arrangement that works for you is nearly as important as finding one that works for your child.

As a final point, I should say that the dichotomy at the heart of the decision tree is perhaps misleading. The choice of childcare doesn't have to be either-or. Looking over the data, to the extent we have any evidence day care is worse, it seems to be worse early on in life—say, in the first year or eighteen months. To the extent day care is better, that seems to be truer later in life—say, after a year or eighteen months. Putting this together could argue for a nanny-type arrangement (or a helpful grandparent, or some combination of the two) early on, followed by day care at a slightly older age.

The Bottom Line

- With any childcare arrangement, quality matters. For day care, in particular, you can use some simple tools to try to do your own quality evaluation.
- On average, more time in day-care centers seems to be associated with slightly better cognitive outcomes and slightly worse behavior outcomes.
- The positive effects of day care present more at older ages, the negative ones more at younger ages.
- Kids in day care get sick more, but develop more immunity.
- Parenting quality swamps childcare choices in its importance, so make sure you pick something that works for you as a parent as well.

11

Sleep Training

Sleep. The elusive, mystical dream of new (and old) parents alike.

Most people are prepared for the first couple of sleepless weeks with a baby; maybe your family is around, or at least you aren't working off a base of exhaustion. But then month 2 comes, and still the baby is sleeping only two hours at a stretch. At some point, the pediatrician tells you, "A baby of this size can sleep for up to six hours at a time." You want to poke them in the eye with a pen.

Now it's month 4. There was one amazing night when the baby slept for four hours, but this has never been repeated. It takes two hours to get her to sleep since you can't put her down in the crib until she has been sleeping for at least an hour in your arms. That's one hour of potential sleep for you, gone. Now it's month 6. Now it's month 8. Now it's starting to seem like your baby just wants to hang out in the middle of the night. And it really does seem like you'll never be rested again.

Of course, this is not everyone's experience. There are people who will tell you their baby slept through the night from three weeks on. In my experienced opinion, most of these people are liars, but I guess it is possible a few are not. And certainly some babies sleep better than others. But the fact is that most babies get up a lot at night, and most parents would prefer not to.

This issue has not gone unnoticed by the marketplace. There are a tremendous number of books on strategies to get your child to sleep better. One academic article on parental approaches to sleep lists forty different books, from *Ready, Set, Sleep: 50 Ways to Get Your Child to Sleep* to *Winning Bedtime Battles*.[1] Even a short Amazon perusal reveals at least twenty, including:

- Weissbluth, *Healthy Sleep Habits, Happy Child*
- Ferber, *Solve Your Child's Sleep Problems*
- Ezzo and Bucknam, *On Becoming Baby Wise*
- Pantley, *The No-Cry Sleep Solution*
- Hogg, *Secrets of the Baby Whisperer*
- Waldburger and Spivack, *The Sleepeasy Solution*
- Mindell, *Sleeping Through the Night*
- Giordano, *The Baby Sleep Solution*
- Turgeon and Wright, *The Happy Sleeper*

These books can be quite compelling. They follow a similar formula: describe some science of sleep (some do this better than others), provide a suggested procedure for increasing sleep, describe many anecdotes from successful users. These anecdotes can be very persuasive. The people in the stories typically have problems *way* worse than yours. And look at them! A few days into the new system and they're sleeping for twelve hours and waking up refreshed!

For the most part, these books each have a particular approach. For example, *Healthy Sleep Habits, Happy Child* outlines a system that involves making sure the baby is fed, diapered, and comfortable before leaving them in their crib, but then allowing them to cry it out. The book contains a lot of details—if you plan to sleep train, you'll want to read at least one of these—and a good portion of it describes the research on why this is a good idea.

Some of the systems are more complex than others. With Finn I briefly attempted one that involved picking him up when he cried, then waiting until he stopped, then immediately putting him back down. Then repeat. I abandoned this after three days; I definitely did not achieve the success of the people in the book. I was so tired, I was probably doing it wrong.

The major distinction among these books is whether they advocate a form of "cry it out." Broadly, "cry it out" refers to any system where you leave the baby in his crib on his own at the start of the night, and sometimes let him fall back to sleep on his own if he wakes at some point during the night. The name refers to the fact that if you do this, your baby will cry some at the start. Modifications include varying whether you check on the baby, the length of time you're willing to let them cry, the length of sleep you are trying to achieve, whether you stay in the room with them (without picking them up), etc.

Ferber is the most well-known advocate of these systems—the word *Ferberize* is sometimes used as a verb to refer to this behavior (i.e., "I am going to Ferberize my baby"), although Weissbluth is increasingly popular and also advocates crying it out.

Alternatives like *The No-Cry Sleep Solution* largely avoid "cry it out," opting instead for systems in which the infant is taught to sleep alone without as much crying. Usually there is some crying anyway (it's a baby, after all).

Of course, there is yet a third solution, advocated more strongly in the attachment-parenting community, that you should not be doing this at all. This philosophy is often linked with William Sears, a Californian doctor with more than thirty parenting books to his name.

Proponents of this philosophy argue, basically, that your infant cries because he needs you, and to let him cry is barbaric. But it goes further than this: attachment parenting advocates co-sleeping as well, meaning there is no need for sleep training of any type since there is no goal of getting the child to sleep alone. Proponents of this point out that if your child is in the bed, you don't really have to get up to deal with them—you just roll over and stick a boob in their mouth and go back to sleep.

If you have decided to keep your infant in the bed with you (see the discussion of co-sleeping in chapter 6), then sleep training (at least early on) is probably not a feasible option. People do try to sleep train older toddlers who share a bed with them, but this is a discussion for another day. But if you are not doing this and your baby is in another room, after getting up every two hours to feed/rock/beg them to sleep, sleep training may begin to seem appealing.

But: Go on the internet, and you'll immediately find a variety of articles detailing the extensive long-term damage sleep training will do to your child. Google "cry it out," and on the first page of results you'll find an article by a PhD psychologist, Darcia Narvaez, entitled "Dangers of 'Crying It Out': Damaging Children and Their Relationships for the Long Term."[2] The article proceeds as you'd expect based on the title. It details the selfish reasons people would choose to do this, and the many long-term psychological issues it could create.

At its core, the concern from the opponents of "cry it out" is that your baby will feel abandoned and, as a result, struggle to form attachments to you, and ultimately to anyone else. It is worth a brief digression on where this idea comes from.

The answer: Romanian orphanages.

In the 1980s, a deep failure of reproductive policy left thousands of infants and children in Romanian orphanages. These children suffered all kinds of tragic deprivations, including limited food, as well as physical and sexual abuse. In addition, they had almost no adult contact as infants and children. They were left in their cribs for years with virtually no human contact, resulting in very late physical development, in addition to mental and psychological costs. Researchers who visited these children found the children could not form bonds with others, and many of them have struggled their whole lives.

This influenced the attachment-parenting philosophy, including views on the use of "cry it out." One of the things visitors noticed in these places was the eerie quiet of the rooms the children were kept in. Infants and babies didn't cry, because they knew no one would come. The argument is that "cry it out" is the same thing: Your baby will stop crying because she knows you will not come, just as the children in these orphanages did. And just as in those settings, her ability to attach to you and others will be forever changed.

This was a terrible and shameful episode that should never have happened. But it is also not comparable to the experience of most infants whose parents use "cry it out" methods. None of these suggest leaving the infant for months without any human contact, nor do they suggest subjecting children to the other types of physical and emotional abuse common in the Romanian orphanage experience.

Obviously, the writers of anti-"cry it out" articles understand this, but in their view, "cry it out" is a continuum. The children left in these orphanages suffered extreme long-term consequences. Children who experience other types of chronic life stress—physical abuse, serious neglect—often have long-term problems. A few nights of sleep training probably will not do that, but who knows whether they endure smaller damages?

Fortunately, the literature does know—at least to some extent—and we can subject the question of whether sleep training is harmful to the data. But before getting into that later in this chapter, it seems useful to start with the basic question of whether sleep training works. Even if you do not think there are long-term consequences of sleep training, it is unpleasant to do—most parents do not like to listen to their children cry. If it doesn't work, it seems like something to avoid. So we'll start there. If the method works, if it has some benefits, we can then move on to the possible risks.

DOES IT WORK?

Good news: yes, this method works for improving sleep.

There are many, many studies on this, employing a variety of related procedures (many of these are randomized trials). A 2006 review covered nineteen studies of the unfortunately named "Extinction" method—the form of "cry it out" in which you leave and do not return—of which seventeen showed improvements in sleep.[3] Another fourteen studies used "Graduated Extinction"—where you come in to check on the baby at increasingly lengthy intervals—and all showed improvements. A smaller number of studies covered "Extinction with Parental Presence"—in which you stay in the room but let the child cry—and these also showed positive effects.

These effects persist through six months or a year in studies that can look this far out. This means that children who are sleep trained are sleeping better (on average) even a year after the training.

These methods do not completely solve all sleep problems from day one. And some children respond better than others, as do some parents. To give an example, in one study of "cry it out" from the 1980s, the authors found that babies in the control group got up four nights a week on average, versus only two nights for babies who were sleep trained.[4] The sleep-trained babies also woke up less frequently on the nights they did get up.

These results are similar to other studies in their magnitudes. Not every baby who is sleep trained will sleep through the night every night, but they do sleep better on average. Getting up four nights a week is significantly worse than getting up two nights.

The bottom line is that there is simply a tremendous amount of evidence suggesting that "cry it out" is an effective method of improving sleep.

It is worth noting that most of these studies—and, indeed, virtually all sleep books—recommend a "bedtime routine" as part of any sleep intervention. There isn't much direct evidence on this—the review refers to it as a "common sense recommendation"—but it is generally included with all intervention approaches. The idea is to have some activities that signal to the baby that it is bedtime: putting on the baby's pajamas, reading them a book, singing some kind of song, turning off the lights. Basically, no one recommends throwing a fully clothed baby in the crib with the lights on, telling them it is bedtime, and closing the door.

BENEFITS

While much of the popular discussion of sleep training focuses on its possible harms, much of the academic literature focuses on its possible benefits, including not only improvements in infant sleep but also benefits to the parents.

Most important, sleep interventions seem to be very successful at reducing maternal depression. To take one example, an Australian study of 328 children randomized half into a sleep-training regime and the other half into a control group. Two and four months later, the authors found that the mothers of babies in the sleep-training arm were less likely to be depressed and more likely to have better physical health. They were less likely to use health services as well.[5]

This finding is consistent across studies. Sleep-training methods consistently improve parental mental health; this includes less depression, higher marital satisfaction, and lower parenting stress.[6] In some cases the effects are very large. One small (non-randomized) study reported that 70 percent of mothers fit the criteria for clinical depression at study enrollment, and only 10 percent after the intervention.[7]

Obviously, we want to think carefully about any possible risks to babies, but the fact that sleep training is good for parents should not be ignored. And sleep is also beneficial to development for babies and kids. Settling into a good sleep routine—one that will ensure longer and higher-quality sleep—could have long-term positive effects for children.

IS "CRY IT OUT" HARMFUL?

"Cry it out" works, helps parents and kids sleep better, and improves parental mood and happiness. Is it harmful for your child?

There are a number of good randomized trials that speak to this. One representative study from Sweden, published in 2004, took ninety-five families and randomized them into a sleep-training regime involving a form of "cry it out."[8] The authors focused on whether behavior during the day was impacted by the nighttime—basically, they asked whether the infants were less attached to their parents during the day as a result of being left to cry during the night.

This particular study found that, in fact, infant security and attachment seemed to *increase* after the "cry it out" intervention. It also found improvements in daytime behavior and eating as reported by the babies' parents. Note that this is the opposite of the concerns raised about "cry it out" methods.

This study is not alone. A 2006 review of sleep-training studies, which included thirteen different interventions, noted the following: "Adverse secondary effects as the result of participating in behaviorally based sleep programs were not identified in any of the studies. On the contrary, infants who participated in sleep interventions were found to be more secure, predictable, less irritable, and to cry and fuss less following treatment."[9] (Translation: Nothing bad happened in any study, and in most cases, the babies seemed happier after sleep training than before.) More recent studies draw the same conclusion.[10]

One interpretation of all these findings is that the babies are better rested, the parents are better rested, and everyone is therefore in a better mood. But this is beyond what is in the data, which doesn't really speak to mechanisms, only to effects.

This evidence focuses on immediate impacts on the infant. But this isn't necessarily the main concern among those who shun "cry it out." Instead, the worry is about longer-term impacts. Yes, the infant cries less— maybe even less during the day—but because they have given up, not because they are happier.

To more fully address this, we need to follow sleep-trained children to older ages to see whether there are long-term risks. This adds to the difficulty of running a randomized trial, of course, since longer-term follow-up is both difficult and expensive. However, we have one example: the same study I discussed on page 177 in the context of sleep-training benefits.

This study was run in Australia, with 328 families recruited when their babies were eight months old. The authors first showed that the intervention improved sleep and lowered parental depression.[11] But they didn't stop there. They returned to evaluate the children a year later and, most notable, five years later, when the children were almost six. In this later follow-up, which included a subset of the original families, the researchers found no difference in any outcomes, including emotional stability and conduct behavior, stress, parent-child closeness, conflict, parent-child attachment, or attachment in general. Basically, the kids who were sleep trained looked exactly like those who were not.[12]

This study—as well as the others I cited earlier and various review articles—does not point to either long- or short-term harms from "cry it out." And it works, and it is good for parents. This paints a pretty pro–"cry it out" picture. But it is not one that everyone agrees with.

A number of academic articles argue against "cry it out" from a theoretical perspective. One good example comes from an article published in 2011 in a journal called *Sleep Medicine Reviews*.[13] The authors of this article presented a case against "cry it out," largely based on the idea that infant crying is intended as a signal of distress, and parents should therefore not be encouraged to ignore it. They draw on the attachment theories cited earlier (i.e., the orphanage literature), and argue that parents who engage in this are ignoring their children's efforts to begin communication with them.

The fact that "cry it out" works is not compelling to these researchers and, indeed, is an indication of harm. As one article in the journal *Sleep* put it, "Is the cessation of crying a 'cure' or is it that the child has 'given up' and is now depressed and has partially withdrawn from the attachment dyad?"[14]

The primary argument offered by this and similar papers is that infant crying is a signal of stress (probably true) and that stress, even over a short period of days or weeks, may have long-term consequences for babies (this is speculative). These authors often point to one particular study to support these stress claims. That study, published in 2012, followed twenty-five infants and their mothers in New Zealand over a five-day inpatient treatment in a sleep lab.[15] The goal of the stay in the lab was to sleep train the infants. Nurses in the study collected data on the stress hormone cortisol in both the babies and their mothers, and were also responsible for putting the infants to sleep, and monitoring the sleep training.

Before the sleep training each day, the babies' and moms' cortisol levels were tested and recorded. This was done again after the infant fell asleep. On the first day, the babies all cried. Their cortisol levels were the same before the training and after they fell asleep. Their mothers' cortisol levels were also the same before the babies cried and after they were asleep. This was the same on the second day.

On the third day, none of the infants cried (see above: sleep training works). However, they showed the same cortisol patterns: equal before bedtime and after they fell asleep. But for the moms, this changed: they had lower cortisol levels in the later period, when the babies weren't crying.

The authors suggested that this presents a problem with sleep training. In particular, they note that after sleep training, the mother's stress levels do not stay in sync with the infant's, which they interpret as possible evidence that the attachment between mother and infant is weakening.

A number of commentators have argued that this is an overinterpretation of the study. For one thing, there is no baseline level of cortisol given, so we actually have no way to know if the babies were even experiencing elevated stress. For another, the study stopped after three days (or at least the data reporting did), so we don't know what happened later.

But even beyond this, it is unclear why differing levels of cortisol for moms and infants after sleep training is a problem. Effectively, this study shows that mothers are more relaxed after sleep training occurs, and that there are no other changes for the infant. This seems like a positive result, not a negative one.

Fundamentally, the argument against sleep training is theoretical. We know that abuse and neglect have long-term consequences, so how can we be sure that four days of a baby crying itself to sleep doesn't? You might think you could look at the data on long-term impacts and note that everything seems fine, but the theoretical counterargument is simply that for some children, this is devastating, and you do not know who those children are.

This argument is nearly impossible to refute. There is no way to prove or disprove it. You'd need a huge sample size, and even then most studies wouldn't be designed to pick up this kind of heterogeneity.

A related argument is that although children may look fine at five or six years old, the damage from sleep training may not manifest until they are adults. Again, very hard to study.

I think it is fair to say that it would be good to have more data—it's always good to have more data! And yes, it is possible that if we had more data, we would find some small negative effects. The studies we have are not perfect.

However, the idea that this uncertainty should lead us to avoid sleep training is flawed. Among other things, you could easily argue the opposite: maybe sleep training is very *good* for some kids—they really need the uninterrupted sleep—and there is a risk of damaging your child by not sleep training. There isn't anything in the data that shows this, but there is similarly nothing to show that sleep training is bad.

You could also argue that the effects of maternal depression on children are long-lasting, and therefore this intervention may have beneficial long-term effects. This seems in many ways more plausible.

You'll have to make a choice about this without perfect data. (This is true of virtually all parenting choices. Blame the parenting researchers!) But it would be a mistake to say, for example, that not sleep training is the "safest option."

Does all this mean you should definitely sleep train? Of course not—every family is different, and you may really not want to let your baby "cry it out." You need to make your own choices, just as with everything else. But if you do want sleep train, you should not feel shame or discomfort about that decision. The data, imperfect as it is, is on your side.

WHICH METHOD, AND WHEN?

Most "cry it out" methods are variants on one of three themes: Extinction—just leave, and do not return; Graduated Extinction—come back at increasingly lengthy intervals; and Extinction with Parental Presence—sit in the room, but do not do anything. Ferber is a proponent of the second, whereas Weissbluth is more in favor of the first.

There is evidence that all three methods work—more evidence, perhaps, on the first two than the third—but relatively little evidence on which works best. On the one hand, some reports seem to find that Graduated Extinction is easier for parents and leads to more consistency; other studies have found it prolongs crying.[16]

The only general principle from these is that consistency is key. Choosing a method—whichever one—and sticking with it increases success. So the most important consideration here is likely what *you* think you can do. Will knowing you can check on the baby help you feel better? Or would you rather just close the door and leave it closed?

This also highlights the importance of having a plan. Sleep training should not be something you decide to do on a whim because your baby is being a jerk today. It should be something you plan—ideally with both parents and caregivers, and perhaps also with your doctor. And once you have a plan, stick to it.

There is relatively little guidance on the appropriate age to start sleep training. Most studies focus on children in the four- to fifteen-month-old period, although these studies tend to recruit people with babies who have been diagnosed with sleep problems, so they are going to be, on average, older. Generally, it will be easier to sleep train a six-month-old than a three-month-old, and probably harder to train a two-year-old. But these methods seem to work on a variety of ages.

What is very important to note is that your sleep-training goals may differ depending on the age of your child. Weissbluth, for example, suggests you can begin sleep training as early as eight or ten weeks. At this age, most babies are *not* able to sleep through the night without eating. You should not expect your two-month-old to sleep for twelve hours, and you similarly shouldn't be frustrated or feel like a failure if they do not. The goal of sleep training a ten-week-old baby is to encourage the baby to fall asleep on their own at the start of the night and then only wake when they are hungry later in the night.

On the other hand, a ten- or eleven-month-old should be able to go through the night without eating, and sleep training babies at that age tends to focus on both their falling asleep on their own and staying asleep through the night.

Put simply, the goal of sleep training is not (despite what some would say) to deprive your child of basic needs like food and diaper changes. It is to encourage their going to sleep independently once those needs are met.

A NOTE ON NAPS

For the most part, the sleep books also suggest that you can use whatever system you are using at night during the day. This includes a version of "cry it out."

There is, however, no research I can identify that specifically focuses on daytime sleep training. There is no particular reason to think that crying during the day would be more or less harmful than crying at night, so on this dimension it is not clear if the lack of specific research is an issue. What is more complicated is the question of whether daytime sleep training will work.

Daytime sleep is more complicated than nighttime sleep. It comes together later (as we talked about in the baby-organization chapter), and it is dropped sooner. Even infants who sleep very well at night have more variable daytime sleeping schedules. All this is to say that sleep training is likely to be more hit-or-miss for naps than at bedtime.

SO, WHAT DID YOU DO?

When Penelope was a baby, we lived in Chicago, and we had a wonderful pediatrician, Dr. Li, who happened to be part of the Weissbluth practice. We never saw Weissbluth himself, but the practice in general was supportive of sleep training. And we did sleep train Penelope, working roughly out of the *Healthy Sleep Habits, Happy Child* playbook.

However, I will say we didn't do the greatest job with consistency. We started with a form of Graduated Extinction—crying with checking—which definitely improved things, but didn't fully work. We had months of on-and-off days of crying, and endless discussions of how long the checking intervals should be, who should do the checking, and so on.

Finally, at one pediatrician visit, we explained our system to Dr. Li, who told us, nicely but firmly, that we should probably cut it out with the checks. When we did this, the sleep training finally took, and Penelope became (and remains) a good sleeper.

I wanted to do a better job with sleep training the second time around. With Finn, we would have a plan—one we had written down, agreed upon, and would stick to.

We used our family task-management software, Asana, for the planning. Jesse created a task—"Finn Sleep Training"—where we could discuss the details back and forth.

(Why, you ask, do you not use email or—heaven forbid—discuss in person? We like to avoid emails for family tasks since they gunk up our work inboxes and it can be hard to find the thread later. And we, at least, have found that it is much more helpful to have discussions like this, especially when opinions abound and emotions run high, in writing rather than in person. It can be easier to fight it out in writing, so everyone gets to quietly think about what they are saying. Then we can save our in-person discussions for such exciting topics as departmental hiring priorities. Fun!)

After some back and forth, we agreed on the following system.

PART 1: BEDTIME/START OF NIGHT

- Finn will go to bed during Penelope's bedtime, around 6:45.
- We will put his pj's on and read him a book as part of the bedtime routine.
- He will nurse, and then we'll put him down in bed.
- *We will not return at all before 10:45 p.m.*

PART 2: OVERNIGHT SCHEDULE

- Will feed Finn the first time he cries after 10:45 p.m.
- After the first feeding, do not respond again until at least 2 hours after the end of each feeding.

Example: If he eats from midnight to 12:30 a.m., then do not respond for another feeding until, at the earliest, 2:30 a.m.

NOTE: THE LONGEST STRETCH OF SLEEP IS EARLY IN THE NIGHT, SO WEISSBLUTH SAYS WE SHOULD RESPOND MORE FREQUENTLY IN THIS PERIOD THAN AT THE START OF THE NIGHT.

PART 3: THE MORNING

- Wake-up is between 6:30 and 7:30 a.m.
- If he is awake at 6:30 we get him up.
- If he is not awake he can sleep until as late as 7:30. At that time we wake him up if he is not up already.

This plan is roughly in the Weissbluth mode. The goal was to encourage Finn to go to sleep on his own at bedtime, but not to deprive him of food. We started this around ten weeks, at which point he was still eating two or three times a night, but we thought he was ready to fall asleep alone at the start of the night.

I did get a successful do-over on this one. Finn was much easier than Penelope—he cried for perhaps twenty-five minutes the first night, a few minutes on the second, and then very little after that. Just to be clear: He did get up (frequently) later in the night after this first stage. He was seven or eight months old before he actually slept through the night.

I think part of our success was having a plan written down. You may not want to be quite so formal, and even if you have a plan, there will likely be some deviation from it—that is okay! But knowing at least in rough terms what you are planning, and agreeing with your partner on it, is likely a good idea.

Part of our success with Finn, we know, was simply because he was an easier baby than Penelope. We were also more experienced parents. Even if you treat your kids exactly the same, they may be different. Some will respond better than others.

Finally, a big part of our success on our second round was having Penelope there.

The great fear during sleep training is that the next time you go see your baby, they will hate you. Your only hope for real success is if you can convince yourself that this is good for your family, and will help you and your baby be better rested. And if you can remember that it will not cause long-term harm.

Of course, this is all hard to remember in the moment. When we were going through this with Finn the first night, he was crying and we were finishing putting Penelope to bed. I was anxious—no matter how convinced you are of the plan, it is very hard to listen to your baby cry. Penelope looked at me—very seriously—and told me, "Mom, whatever you do, you can't go in. He needs to learn to sleep on his own. We have to help him do that."

In the presence of a child who was sleep trained and obviously does not hate you, it is hard to hold on to your fear.

The Bottom Line

- "Cry it out" methods are effective at encouraging nighttime sleep.
- There is evidence that using these methods improves outcomes for parents, including less depression and better general mental health.
- There is no evidence of long- or short-term harm to infants; if anything, there may be some evidence of short-term benefits.
- There is evidence of success for a wide variety of specific methods, and little to distinguish between them.
  - The most important thing is consistency: choose a method you can stick with, and stick with it.

Beyond the Boobs:
Introducing Solid Food

Gideon Lack is a researcher at King's College London. He studies allergies in kids, especially allergies to peanuts. At some point, perhaps through discussions with colleagues in Israel, Dr. Lack got the impression that peanut allergies were much less common among children in Israel than in the UK. So in 2008 he published a paper testing this theory. Using a questionnaire, covering about five thousand children in each location and focusing on Jewish children in both Israel and the UK, he found that school-age children in the UK were about ten times more likely to be allergic to peanuts than children in Israel.[1] Almost 2 percent of the children in the UK were allergic, versus just 0.2 percent of the Israeli children.

In the paper reporting these findings, Dr. Lack and his colleagues went beyond just showing the prevalence differences. They actually speculated as to why the differences existed: specifically, early peanut exposure. Children in Israel are more commonly exposed to peanuts early in life—there is a popular peanut-based early childhood snack called

Bamba—and the researchers argued that this exposure may be the cause of lower incidence of peanut allergies in Israeli children.

The careful reader will know this type of claim is exactly the kind of thing that drives me crazy. A huge number of things differ between Israel and the UK! These issues are by no means fully addressed by using only Jewish children in the UK. An obvious difference is diagnosis rate—what if even mild peanut allergies are diagnosed in the UK, and only severe ones in Israel? Since the data is based only on a questionnaire, we have no way to verify the allergy or how bad it is.

Gideon Lack might have stopped there, and we'd be left with a vaguely interesting fact and some unsatisfying speculation about why, but he didn't. He pursued this idea using a much more convincing method: a randomized controlled trial.

In the years following their initial findings, Lack and his colleagues recruited a cohort of about seven hundred babies between four and eleven months old and randomized them into a peanut exposure group and a non-exposure group. Parents of children in the exposure group were told to expose their kids to a dose of peanuts—about 6 grams a week—in the form of either the Israeli snack Bamba or regular peanut butter. Parents of children in the other group were told to avoid peanuts.

The researchers selected a group of children who were more likely to have peanut allergies than the general population—this was important to make sure they could draw strong conclusions even with a relatively small sample size—and they also divided the sample into children who had no sensitivity to peanuts at baseline and those who showed some sensitivity. This let them look at these effects overall, and in children who were more prone to allergy. The kids were, of course, closely monitored for any adverse reactions.

The researchers finally published their findings in 2015 in the *New England Journal of Medicine*.[2] The results—I put them in a graph on page 190—are striking. Children who were exposed to peanuts were far less likely to be allergic to them at the age of five than children who were not. In the group that didn't get peanuts, 17 percent of children were allergic to peanuts at age five. (Remember, this figure is higher than it would be in the general population because of the way the researchers selected their sample.) However, only 3 percent of the children who were given peanuts were allergic.

Since the study was randomized, there was no reason other than the peanut exposure that allergy rates would be different. And these differences showed up in both the high- and low-allergy-risk groups.

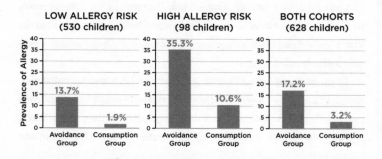

This is a striking finding, to say the least. It suggests that exposing children to peanuts early helps them avoid peanut allergies. The finding is especially notable as it suggests that the standard advice parents were given about peanuts up to this point was entirely wrong. (With Penelope, we were told to wait until she was a year old to introduce peanuts.) This advice was given especially to people whose children were at higher risk for allergy.[3]

It is not an exaggeration to say this advice has made things worse and, indeed, may be largely responsible for the increase in peanut allergies over the past twenty years. The fact that your kid has to bring SunButter to school? That may well be the fault of bad public health advice.

In the wake of these peanut findings, the recommendations about exposure have changed completely. Early exposure to peanuts is now the normal recommendation, especially for children at risk for an allergy. The hope is that with wider dissemination and use of these updated recommendations, there will be fewer life-threatening peanut allergies. And we'll have Gideon Lack to thank. Of course, this does highlight the problems with basing your initial recommendations on little or no evidence.

Peanut timing is not the only recommendation that you'll hear about food. The American Academy of Pediatrics (among other sources) has whole websites devoted to transitioning your child to eating solid foods. For the most part, there is little real evidence behind these recommendations.

The AAP recommendations echo the traditional Western way to introduce your children to food. This begins, between four and six months, with either rice cereal or oatmeal. You feed your child with a spoon. Make sure to take some adorable pictures to send to the grandparents! These will also be helpful at your child's wedding.

Then, a few days or a week later, you introduce fruits and vegetables, one variety at a time, every three days. The standard advice is to do veggies first so kids do not learn fruit tastes better. A month or so after that, you introduce meat. All of this is in a pureed form and fed to your baby with a spoon.

With Penelope we followed this exactly. I made a brief foray into making my own baby food, which I gave up almost immediately. I did invest in the world's largest supply of Earth's Best organic baby food. We actually had a special closet devoted to the jars. When Penelope finally aged out of it, we still had whole pallets of chicken and sweet potato "Step 2" jars.

Eventually, you introduce foods the kid can pick up with their hands. This would include, say, Cheerios and rice puffs. Gradually, around a year or so, you phase out the pureed food. (In case you are wondering, yes, a food pantry will take those jars you have stacked in the closet.)

There is certainly nothing wrong with these recommendations, per se. They have worked for many people for many years.

And there is some reasoning behind this approach. Before four months, your baby is unlikely to be able to eat solid food—the skill is fundamentally different from nursing or drinking from a bottle—and there is no reason to give them anything other than breast milk. There is also a concern about filling their stomach with foods that, unlike breast milk and formula, do not give them the appropriate nutrients for their age. This gives you part of the timing recommendation.

You start with rice cereal because it is flavorless, and you can therefore mix it with breast milk or formula so your kid is more likely to eat it. These cereals are also iron fortified, which is helpful if you're nursing, since this is an age at which breast milk may no longer provide enough iron.

The delay between food introductions is to see if any food causes an allergy. If you feed your kid strawberries and eggs and tomatoes and wheat all in a single day and they have an allergic reaction, it will be hard to know what the source is.

All these arguments are logical, but there isn't much testing of the specifics. At best, I would therefore describe these recommendations as logic based rather than evidence based.

For example, there is no evidence for the order of food introductions. If you'd like to start with carrots or prunes rather than rice cereal, I can find no reason in the published evidence not to. Sure, maybe your baby will be more comfortable with rice cereal, but carrots are actually objectively tastier. Finn thought those cereals were a joke. The only rice cereal he ever ate was congee at our favorite Chinese restaurant.

Similarly, there is some sensibility behind the idea of waiting between food introductions. Nearly all allergies are caused by one of a few foods—milk, eggs, peanuts, and tree nuts—and it's sensible not to introduce these foods all at the same time. But most people are not allergic to most things. Yes, you can have an allergy to peas, but this is very uncommon. This doesn't mean there is anything wrong with the every-three-days plan, and based on other evidence that kids need to try a food a few times before they like it, there may be a reason to focus on adding new foods one at a time. On the other hand, if you plan to introduce all the foods to your kid before they are one, you'll have to speed up at some point.

This discussion relates to small modifications around the traditional food introduction plan. But some people go further with this and question the very approach of spoon-feeding purees in the first place. An alternative, which has grown in popularity in recent years, is referred to as "baby-led weaning." In this practice, instead of introducing pureed foods and feeding the kid with a spoon, you wait until they are old enough to pick up foods on their own and then have them more or less eat what your family eats.

I used this approach with Finn. I wish I could say it was because I belatedly discovered a large evidence base suggesting it was better. In fact, it was that I could not bear the thought of another closet full of jars. Baby-led weaning involves just giving your child the food you are eating. This seemed great! I was already producing that food. I was all for signing up for an easier approach that preserved my closet space.

Advocates of baby-led weaning do not typically focus on the lazy-parenting benefits. Instead, they cite benefits to your child: infants learn to regulate the amount of food they eat, leading to less incidence of overweight or obesity; they show acceptance of a wide variety of foods; and you have better family mealtime experiences.

Evidence backing these claims is, however, limited.[4] A main issue is that the kinds of parents who are likely to try this differ from those who use a more traditional feeding structure. They tend to be higher income, better educated, more likely to sit together at family meals, etc. These factors also relate to mealtime experience and diet quality, making it hard to separate out the role of the food introduction system.

The best evidence we have is from one (small) randomized trial of two hundred families.[5] The results support some of the claims about baby-led weaning, but not all. Parents reported less food fussiness, and the infants in the baby-led weaning group were more likely to eat with their family. They were also likely to be breastfed longer, and the introduction of food was pushed later (i.e., to around six months rather than four).

On the other hand, this study did not find any differences in whether children were overweight or obese by the age of two, and they didn't find any differences in the nutrients the children consumed or their total calorie intake. The researchers noted that this was hard to measure given the smearing around of food. The kids did eat slightly differently—the baby-led-weaning group was more likely to have meat and salt, for example—but these differences didn't go in any systematic direction.

One of the main concerns with this approach is that it could lead to choking, if infants are unable to swallow big pieces of things. The study showed that it was no more common in the baby-led-weaning group than the traditional spoon-feeding group. Choking is, however, reasonably common in all babies, and people in the study were encouraged not to introduce foods that presented significant choking hazards. A four-month-old shouldn't have large pieces of hard fruit, baby-led weaning or not.

This study followed two hundred people; clearly, learning detailed answers to these questions would require a lot more than that. If you do want to try baby-led weaning, there is nothing in the evidence to say it is a bad idea. If you do not, there is also nothing compelling to say you should go out and do it.

A final note on timing: There is some debate about the right time to introduce solid foods and, in particular, a question of whether introducing solids too early will lead to obesity later. What is the reason to wait for four months at all? Should you really be waiting for six months, or longer? The reasons to wait until four months are largely physiological—babies really cannot eat before this—but waiting longer than that doesn't seem like it matters. There is some correlation between the timing of food introduction and childhood obesity, but it seems to be due to other factors, like parental weight and diet.[6]

DOES WHAT YOU FEED YOUR KIDS MATTER?

Deciding whether to start with purees is one thing, but there is a more important question here: What, exactly, should you be feeding your child? The bottom line is that more or less everyone on the planet eats, and they more or less all eat solid food, so regardless of how you introduce foods, you're likely to end up with a child who eats something.

There is no guarantee, however, that your child will like a wide variety of foods, will eat healthily, and will be willing to try new things. Perhaps it isn't difficult to produce a child who will eat chicken nuggets and hot dogs, but how do you end up with one who loves sautéed kale and kimchi with squid? Or at least one who will try them?

Let's acknowledge: this issue may not be important to everyone. You may care that your child is willing to eat some vegetables, but you may not particularly care if they are picky or not. There is nothing wrong with a child who eats only broccoli and pasta, as long as that works for your family. Going further, you may not care if the child eats only pasta, figuring they'll get into broccoli when they grow up. You will need to think more carefully, in this case, about how your child will get the necessary vitamins, but otherwise this is not obviously problematic.

How much you care about this is likely to depend on how your family eats. For a while I was making two dinners—one for Penelope and a later one for us—and it got to be too much. Ultimately, we altered both what we ate and what she ate so we could eat together. But many people are fine with the system of two dinners.

Let's assume, however, that you do care about promoting a "healthy diet." The good news is that there is plenty of research on this question. The bad news is that a lot of it is not very good.

Consider a paper from 2017 that got a lot of media attention.[7] The authors followed 911 children from age nine months to six years and related their early diet to their later diet. They found that children who ate a varied diet—and in particular those who consumed a wide variety of fruits and vegetables—at nine months were also more likely to eat a varied diet with vegetables at age six.

The researchers concluded that tastes are formed early, and it is therefore important to expose children to a variety of foods early in life.

This is certainly one possible explanation for the results. But it is by no means the most likely one. A much more plausible explanation is that the parents who feed their children vegetables at age one are also likely to feed them vegetables at age six. This is just a very basic causality problem, and it is difficult to learn anything here.

However, we can get some clues about the true underlying relationships from smaller, more indirect studies.

Consider the following quite neat example. Researchers recruited a group of moms and randomized them into a "high-carrot" or "low-carrot" diet during pregnancy and lactation. The high-carrot moms were drinking a lot of carrot juice.

When their children were ready for rice cereal, the researchers offered them (the babies, not the moms) cereal made with water, or one flavored with carrots. The kids whose moms had eaten more carrots were more likely to prefer the carrot cereal (as evidenced by their consumption and their facial expressions, and presumably also whether they picked up the dish and threw it on the floor).[8] This suggests that flavor exposure—in this case, thorough the placenta and through breast milk—affects whether children are receptive to new flavors.

Related to this, once children are starting to eat solid foods, there is randomized evidence that repeated exposure to a food—say, giving kids pears every day for a week—increases their liking of it. This works for fruits, but also for vegetables, even bitter ones.[9] It reinforces the idea that children can get used to different flavors and that they like familiar ones.

This shouldn't be too surprising. People eat differently in different cultures, and we know people continue to express preferences for the foods they ate as a child, even if they move to another location.[10]

Putting this together, on one hand, from a global public health perspective, I would be extremely hesitant to conclude that lack of exposure to vegetables at age one was the main problem with older children's diets. The problem is more likely to be with the foods kids are offered at both ages. On the other hand, from the standpoint of an individual parent, if you want your child to eat a variety of foods, this suggests it is beneficial to expose them—repeatedly—to these flavors.

However, even if you eat all kinds of weird stuff while breastfeeding, and carefully expose your child to Brussels sprouts for weeks on end, they may still end up being somewhat picky about their food. Researchers classify this pickiness into two groups: food neophobia (fear of new foods) and picky/fussy eating, in which the child just doesn't like a lot of different foods.

Before getting into these, and how you might fix them (hard), you should know that most kids become more picky around two and then slowly grow out of it in their elementary school years. This is sometimes a surprise to parents—your eighteen-month-old eats like a horse, then all of a sudden around two, they start being very selective and just generally not eating much. I have sat at many a dinner where one of my kids has taken one bite and said, "I'm done!"

This change can lead to unrealistic expectations from parents about how much their toddler and young child will eat. As a review article from 2012 notes, "The majority of children between one and five years of age who are brought in by their parents for refusing to eat are healthy and have an appetite that is appropriate for their age and growth rate."[11] The article goes on to note that the most useful treatment for this problem is parental counseling, not anything to do with the child. Thanks for the judgment, researchers.

This suggests that even if your child doesn't eat that much some of the time, you probably shouldn't be overly concerned, but it doesn't answer the question of how you can treat or avoid general pickiness. This is a topic of some research interest. One study I like a lot followed sixty families of kids aged twelve to thirty-six months as they tried introducing a new food. The families videotaped their dinner interactions for a night so researchers could study what seemed to influence the new food adoption.[12]

This study reported what parents actually do rather than what they say they do. This is good, since none of us is especially good at reporting our actual behavior. The primary finding relates to how parents talk about the new food. Kids are more likely to try to eat it with what researchers call "autonomy-supportive prompts"—things like "Try your hot dog" or "Prunes are like big raisins, so you might like them." In contrast, they are less likely to try things if parents use "coercive-controlling prompts"—things like "If you finish your pasta, you can have ice cream" or "If you won't eat, I'm taking away your iPad!!"

Other studies show that parental pressure to try new foods or to eat in general is associated with more food refusal, not less.[13] These studies also show that food refusals are more common in families where parents offer an alternative. That is, if your kid doesn't eat broccoli and then you offer him chicken nuggets instead, he may learn that this is always the reward for not eating new foods. This problem is exacerbated by parents' concern that their child isn't eating enough (which, see above, is probably not true).

Putting this together leads to some general advice: offer your very young child a wide variety of foods, and keep offering them even if the child rejects them at first. As they get a little older, do not freak out if they don't eat as much as you expect, and keep offering them new and varied foods. If they won't eat the new foods, don't replace the foods with something else that they do like or will eat. And don't use threats or rewards to coerce them to eat.

This advice is easy to give but it can be hard to take. It is frustrating to sit at a meal that you know to be delicious with a four-year-old who screams that they hate it and will not eat anything. I don't have a great solution for this, other than earplugs.

I also tried to train Finn to say "I don't care for pot roast" rather than "I HATE POT ROAST," since it at least sounds more polite, even if still combined with pushing the plate away and putting on an angry pouty face. (Parenting: It's a long game.)

All this discussion is predicated on the assumption that your child doesn't actually have a problem with weight gain or nutrition. If you are worried, this is what the pediatrician is for—they can check on weight gain, malnutrition, vitamins, and so on. For children who are malnourished, there is a whole other set of guidelines, most of which are more intense and involved, for increasing eating.

ALLERGENS

The story at the start of this chapter gives a sense of how the recommendations for peanuts have changed: introduce early, not later. What the story doesn't convey is whether this translates more generally to allergenic foods, and exactly how you are supposed to introduce them.

On the first question, the answer is probably yes. The vast majority of allergies result from eight food types: milk, peanuts, eggs, soy, wheat, tree nuts, fish, and shellfish. The incidence of these allergies has grown over time, perhaps as a result of better hygiene (so less allergen exposure early on), and clearly due in part to a lack of early introduction.

Milk, eggs, and peanuts make up a large share even of these. We covered the peanut evidence earlier. Other research suggests a similar mechanism is at work for eggs and milk.[14] The evidence on milk isn't as convincing as the other two, but perhaps only because large studies have not yet been released.

All this points to the possible importance of introducing all these allergens early—probably as early as four months. (Milk can be introduced in the form of yogurt or cheese.)

Importantly, although the language here is about "introduction," these studies include regular exposure as well. It is not enough to have your kid try peanut butter or eggs. You need to actually keep giving it to them regularly.

Which leads to the question: How?

This is a setting in which going slowly is a good idea. Try a little bit at first—only one allergenic food in a given day—and see how they react. If nothing, give them a little bit more. And so on until you get up to a normal amount.

And then keep these foods in the rotation.

This is a lot, especially since most babies don't really eat much food anyway. To consistently expose them to peanuts and yogurt and eggs on top of everything else (what about the peas?) requires some logistical work. If you are daunted, and especially if you're very concerned about these issues, there are some (new) products that contain powdered forms of these foods and are meant to be mixed with breast milk, formula, or cereals.

OTHER FORBIDDEN FOODS

Beyond allergens, there are a few other foods on the "forbidden foods" list: cow's milk, honey, choking hazards, and sugar-sweetened beverages. Do these belong there?

The last one is obviously not just about infancy. Soda is strongly discouraged for infants and children (and adults). Your six-month-old does not need a Coke. Juice is more controversial (and, indeed, I recall a childhood dominated by orange juice), but generally, young children should have formula, breast milk, or (once they start eating solid foods) water. Whole fruits or fruit purees are preferable to fruit juice.

Choking hazards—nuts, whole grapes, hard candies—are also to be avoided, for obvious reasons. Babies and toddlers do choke, and these foods are more likely to lead to choking. Grapes are okay in pieces, nuts are okay in nut-butter form, and hard candies are not recommended for other reasons.

Cow's milk is probably the most complicated recommendation, partly because it interacts with the allergen issues above. It is important to introduce some milk-based foods—yogurt, cheese—to avoid allergies. But milk itself is forbidden.

The concern is that cow's milk is not a complete infant nutrition system, and if your infant drinks a lot of milk, it will restrict formula or breast milk intake. In particular, infants who have cow's milk as their primary milk source are more likely to be iron deficient.[15] The evidence says only that you shouldn't replace formula or breast milk with cow's milk. As an addition to, say, oatmeal or cereal, it isn't a problem.

Finally, honey. The concern with honey is that it could lead to infant botulism. Infant botulism is a serious disease—basically, a toxin interferes with neurological functions, including affecting the infant's ability to breathe. It is most common under the age of six months and it is treatable, with a very high success rate. Still, the treatment is not easy: the baby typically needs to be hooked up to a breathing machine for a few days until they are able to breathe on their own again.

The toxin that causes this, *Clostridium botulinum*, is found in soil and elsewhere, including in honey. This, combined with the fact that there were multiple case reports from the 1970s and '80s in which infants who developed botulism had consumed honey, led to the recommendation against honey through the first year of life (sometimes even two or three).

The question of how important honey is as a source of botulism is an open one, though. Although the ban on honey has been widely publicized over the past decades, there has been basically no change in the rate of infant botulism.[16] This suggests that other sources of botulism are more important in practice. So maybe this is overkill, but the downsides of avoiding honey are also limited.

VITAMIN SUPPLEMENTATION

People spend a lot of time telling you how perfect breast milk is, how it's the most amazing food on the planet and contains everything your baby needs! Then, in pretty much the next breath, they hand you a bottle of vitamin D drops and tell you that, actually, breast milk doesn't have enough vitamin D and you'd better remember to give your kid these drops every day, or they might get rickets.

I would describe remembering these drops as a "challenge" for our family. Many a yelled conversation across the house concerned whether someone had given the drop or not that day. The days blur. Was it yesterday, or three weeks ago?

Perhaps we should consider ourselves lucky that Penelope and Finn did not get rickets.

Then again, perhaps this risk is overblown.

The general wisdom of vitamin supplementation (for anyone—adults, children, babies) is complicated. It is true that if you are deficient in particular vitamins, it can cause serious problems. Vitamin D deficiency causes rickets. Vitamin C deficiency famously causes scurvy, as was first recognized in sailors who went months without eating any fresh vegetables or fruit. However, if you eat a typical varied diet—even one that's pretty unhealthy by many standards—you are very unlikely to be seriously deficient in any of these vitamins.

Your toddler or young child does not generally need a multivitamin (no Flintstones gummies for them). If they eat only a *very* limited diet, it is possible a multivitamin would be necessary, but this would be unusual. Even a child who seems like a very picky eater will be getting enough vitamins to sustain them. A baby who is breastfed will get most vitamins this way as well.

The two possible exceptions to this are vitamin D and iron.

Vitamin D is not present in many foods, and is not present in high concentrations in breast milk. People do get vitamin D through sun exposure, but since many of us live in houses in cold places and not on the savanna, sun exposure isn't always consistent.

As a result, a lot of infants and children are considered deficient in vitamin D. This could be as much as a quarter or more of white children, and higher among children of color (darker skin lowers vitamin D absorption from the sun).[17] Deficiency here is defined as having a blood concentration of vitamin D below some cutoff level.

What is less clear is whether this really has much actual health impact. Relatively few studies have looked at the actual *outcomes* associated with vitamin D, like bone growth. In two that did—very small randomized trials of supplementation—there were no impacts on bone growth or bone health, even though supplementation did increase the concentrations of vitamin D in babies.[18]

This isn't to say you shouldn't use vitamin D supplements. And certainly rickets does occur, primarily in developing countries with serious nutritional limits. But it does suggest that if you miss a day here or there, you shouldn't panic.

If you are very uncomfortable directly supplementing your baby, there is evidence that if you are breastfeeding, high levels of supplementation for Mom will increase her vitamin D concentration and accomplish a similar goal.[19]

Breastfed infants are also sometimes iron deficient, which can cause anemia. Breast milk is low in iron. Iron supplementation is not commonly recommended, unless the infant actually shows signs of anemia, and iron is present in rice cereal, so once your kid starts eating, this problem diminishes. Also, anemia rates are improved by delayed cord cutting (see part 1), which is a lot easier than supplementation.

All this supplementation applies to breastfed infants. Formula contains iron and vitamin D, along with the rest of the vitamins. So if you use formula even some of the time, your child is unlikely to have these issues.

The Bottom Line

- Early exposure to allergens reduces incidences of food allergies.
- Kids take time to get used to new flavors, so it is valuable to keep trying a food even if they reject it at first, and early exposure to varying flavors increases acceptance.
- There is not much evidence behind the traditional food-introduction recommendations; no need to do rice cereal first if you do not want to.
- Baby-led weaning doesn't have magical properties (at least not based on what we know now), but there is also no reason not to do it if you want to.
- Vitamin D supplementation is reasonable, but don't freak out about missing a day here and there.

From Baby to Toddler

B abies are exhausting in many ways—they don't sleep, they can't tell you what they want, they eat all the time on an unpredictable schedule. When you have an infant or a four-month-old, you may look forward to the time when your child can eat dinner at the table and tell you what they want.

Once realized, though, this is not always all it's cracked up to be. Take the battle of the socks. With a baby, it can be hard to find socks that do not fall off. But it's easy to put the socks on! They are happy to have them; it's easy to manipulate them. With a baby, rarely do you spend time thinking about getting ready for the day early so as to have time for socks.

Not so with a toddler. "Time for socks and shoes!" you say, eleven minutes before you need to leave the house. "NO! I don't WANT socks! I don't WANT them." Foot stamping, face scrunched up. Arms may be folded in anger pose.

"Let's put on your socks." Wrestling.

"AHHHHH!!!! NOOOO!!!!!"

"If you don't let me put on your socks, I'll have to get Dad to come help."

"NO SOCKS. NOOOO SOCKS!!!!!"

"Sweetie, can you help me with him?" Second parent arrives, holds kid still.

Socks are on. Great! You go looking for shoes. Return. Child has taken off socks, is wearing no socks, just an evil grin. Has also removed pants.

Toddlers are a new ball game. They are funny, playful, exciting to be around. But they also bring resistance. And at the same time, there are more things you are trying to accomplish, things that you need their help with. Sleep training, vaccination—you can do these without your child's cooperation. Potty training, not so much. You can set up a system, you can have stickers, M&M's, a special potty video. But ultimately, your child will have to decide to use the toilet. It's just a fact: you cannot force someone to poop.

Parenting a toddler also seems somehow more consequential than parenting a baby. As you see your child's personality come through, you also start to see what they will struggle with. And you, all of a sudden, face choices—like screen time, or what kind of preschool to send them to—that seem like they may follow your child forever. On top of this, add the issue of discipline, which, suddenly, you have to think about, and it adds up to a much more complex parenting problem.

As your child ages, evidence-based approaches to parenting become more challenging. The more variation across children, the more difficult it is to pull strong conclusions out of data. Heterogeneity across kids means that what works for one kid might not work for another, and if you estimate an effect of some approach on average, you may get nothing, even if it works really well for some kids.

There are, however, some general principles to learn. In this part of the book, I'll also talk a bit about milestones—physical, which you'll see some of in the first year, and language-oriented, which come later. Most of us worry, at least sometimes, whether our kids are developing normally. *Why isn't my daughter crawling or walking or running? Why does my sixteen-month-old just use "da-da" for everything?* There aren't likely any decisions about this, but knowing something about the data can relax even the most neurotic of us.

Unfortunately, I have found nothing in the data to address the sock problem. I am holding out hope for technological progress that will produce a sock you can lock onto your child's leg. Stay tuned.

Early Walking, Late Walking:
Physical Milestones

My friend Jane's son was born three months after Penelope. Once they got a bit older—five, six, seven—you'd never notice this age difference at all, but early on, it was hard to believe that was true. When Benjamin was born, Penelope seemed like a giant. When he was a floppy six-week-old infant, she was four and a half months old, well on her way toward being a real, solid baby.

But then came walking. At a year, like the average kid, Benjamin got up and started toddling around. Not Penelope. By the time he was walking, she was fifteen months old and seemed to show no inclination. It is sometimes easy to ignore the way your children differ from the average, but it's made much harder if you see the average all the time.

At Penelope's fifteen-month well-child visit, the ever-calming Dr. Li told me not to worry that she wasn't walking. "If she's not walking by eighteen months," she said, "we'll call in early intervention. But don't worry! She'll figure it out." Early intervention is an excellent government program designed to intervene at young ages to help kids with developmental delays—physical or mental. This is a hugely valuable program to have access to, but still, I did not like the suggestion that we were approaching it.

I tried to explain to Penelope how to walk; she didn't care. I tried to provide incentives, which really was going off the deep end.

And then, about two weeks after the doctor visit, Penelope walked. Just like it was no big deal. Perhaps because she was so old by the time she learned, she never fell down much, either, just went from crawling around to walking normally in a day or two. And then I promptly forgot about my fear that she would never walk and moved on to other neuroses. (There are always more neuroses around the corner when you're parenting.)

I don't think my experience was unique. In the moment, physical milestones—sitting, crawling, walking, running—take on an outsize importance. I have many notes from the first months of Penelope's life about her rolling ability (very early rolling to the left, but poor rolling to the right). Things like head control are among the first means we have to evaluate how our kids are doing.

Failure to achieve these milestones at the time we expect, therefore, tends to worry parents. I think part of the issue is the focus on average ages—as in, "Most children walk around one year." This is true, but it misses the fact that there is a wide *distribution* in what is typical.

We are used to thinking about these distributions in, say, our child's weight. The average one-year-old weighs 23 pounds, but there are some much smaller and some larger. When you go to the pediatrician for your one-year visit, they'll actually tell you something like, "Your child is at the twenty-fifth percentile for weight."

In the case of milestones—physical, and language development—we don't really talk about distributions. I'm not sure why not; could be lack of data or an unwillingness to assign percentiles in these areas. But whether we discuss them, these distributions are there. And even just knowing this may relax you a bit. It's true that the average age of walking is a year, but having a kid who walks somewhat earlier or later than this one-year average is also totally fine in the same way it's totally fine for your child to be at the 25th (or the 75th) percentile of weight.

So why do we pay attention to this at all? Why do pediatricians evaluate motor skills? There is good reason to do it, but the goal is to detect children who are outside the normal range of the distribution. In particular, pediatricians are looking for kids who are very delayed. Children who are very delayed on early milestones—head control, rolling over—are more likely (not very likely, just *more* likely) to have serious developmental issues.

Some of these issues will also manifest in cognitive or behavioral problems, but we do not see evidence of delays in these areas until kids are much older. There is some literature showing that children with serious early motor delays also show some lower spatial skills in later childhood,[1] and perhaps even have lower reading test scores as middle-age adults.[2] For this reason, detecting early motor delays is a pediatric focus.[3]

There are also some particular diseases or conditions that motor delays can signal.

The primary one is cerebral palsy (CP), which, broadly, is a term for developmental problems caused by very early damage to the nervous system. This affects 1.5 to 3 children in 1,000, meaning it is rare but common enough to be something many pediatricians see in normal practice (these rates are much lower for full-term babies with nontraumatic births). In the past it was believed that CP was exclusively a result of injuries at birth, but more recent evidence suggests prenatal conditions may also have an effect on whether a child is born with CP.[4]

Cerebral palsy isn't a disease—like a virus or cancer—or a genetic defect. It's a term to describe motor issues that result from nervous system injury. The issues resulting from CP vary widely—it can affect different limbs or body parts, and be more or less severe. At birth, doctors are likely to know if babies are at higher risk for CP—due to birth trauma, prematurity, or other risk factors—but a definitive diagnosis typically cannot be made at birth. Instead, CP is typically recognized later when motor development is abnormal. More severe cases can be detected early—at four to six months— but less severe cases may take a year or more to become apparent. Careful evaluation of babies for motor delays is helpful in increasing the chance of early detection, which can in turn lead to earlier intervention.

The other group of conditions that may be detected this way are progressive neurological diseases. These are extremely rare. Muscular dystrophy is the most common, but it affects just 0.2 in 1,000 births. The others are even less common. Given their progressive nature, these are also more difficult to detect early on; still, they are one of the things pediatricians are looking for.

Motor delays are also common in some conditions that you'd know about at birth. Spina bifida (a birth defect in which the body fails to close over the spinal cord), for example, or a genetic condition like Down syndrome. Motor development is carefully monitored for children in this group, but we do not expect these conditions to be detected by motor development alone.

When you see your pediatrician for a well visit (which will happen many, many times in the first three years), they'll be looking for signs of these serious motor delays. But what signs, exactly, and how?

First, at any visit, your doctor will poke around at the baby, see about their muscle development, do various baby manipulations (your baby will not like this). They'll look for good reflexes, for good movement "quality." This is an important part of the evaluation, although pretty hard to quantify (and extremely difficult to evaluate on your own).

In addition, doctors will look for some basic developmental milestones at each visit. Here are some examples from the 9-, 18-, and 30- or 36-month visits.

Visit	Milestones
9 months	Rolling both sides, sitting with support, motor symmetry, grasping and transferring objects between hands.
18 months	Sitting, standing, and walking independently; grasping and manipulating small objects.
30 months	Subtle gross motor errors, looking for loss of previous skills (marker of progressive disease).

The 9- and 18-month milestones are the most crucial here; by 30 months, most major issues have been well identified, and doctors are looking for smaller things.

Nearly all children will have achieved these milestones by these points. Typically, developing babies roll over between 3 and 5 months; if they have not rolled over by 9 months, that is definitely outside the normal. Similarly, although typical development calls for walking between 8 and 17 months—with an average of 12 months—looking at 18 months catches children who are outside the norm.[5]

Setting up formal assessment times is valuable to make sure children with delays are not missed, but a good pediatrician will be evaluating your child's motor development at all visits, and they'll be looking for places where your child is out of the normal range on any particular milestone, or especially on two or more.

What are these normal ranges? For that, we can go to the data. The World Health Organization, using data from six countries, calculated the range of the 1st percentile to 99th percentile for each of a variety of outcomes among healthy children. The children they studied do not have diagnosed motor issues, so their argument is that this can be seen as the range of normal development.[6]

Milestone	Range
Sitting without support	3.8 months to 9.2 months
Standing with assistance	4.8 months to 11.4 months
Crawling (5% of kids never do)	5.2 months to 13.5 months
Walking with help	5.9 months to 13.7 months
Standing alone	6.9 months to 16.9 months
Walking alone	8.2 months to 17.6 months

From this data, we see the logic for Dr. Li's suggestion that we wait for 18 months before panicking about walking, and we see the very wide normal ranges on almost all of these. Standing alone, for example, occurs any time between 7 and 17 months. This is an eternity in baby time!

Your doctor will be very focused—correctly—on the upper ends of these ranges. But what if your kid is walking really early—like, at 7 months? Does this mean they are going to be an amazing athlete? And what if they're at the older end of the normal range—doomed to being picked last for the kickball team?

There is, in fact, very little evidence on the long-term impacts of late walking. Virtually all children—indeed, even the vast majority of those who are delayed—do end up walking and running. If you ask, "Does early walking predict walking?" the answer will be, "No, everyone walks."

When it comes to being an elite athlete, there is just nothing. I don't know if it is just that researchers are not interested in predicting elite athletic performance. Perhaps the issue is that even if there were some relationship, the outcome is so unlikely, we'd never see it in the data. The Olympics, we find, are just not a realistic goal for most people. Thanks, data.

There is simply nothing in the data that would make us think that earlier walking or standing or rolling or head raising is associated with any later outcomes. Looking for delays is a good idea; looking for exceptionalism, or worrying about a child who is at the end of the normal range, is probably not.

ILLNESS

Although not technically a milestone, baby's first cold is definitely a moment for a parent. A bad one. Then there is baby's second cold, baby's third cold, and on and on.

As the parent of a young child, you will spend the period from October to April drowning in a lake of snot. To many of us, it may seem that our child has a cold, or possibly some other illness, literally all the time. If you have two children or, god forbid, more than two, the winter months are a haze of repeated illnesses: you, kid 1, kid 2, your partner, back to kid 2, now kid 1 again. Usually there's a dose of stomach flu somewhere in the middle (you all get that, obviously).

This can naturally leave you wondering, *Is this normal? Is everyone else spending their life savings on tissues with lotion, too?*

Basically, yes.

Kids younger than school age get an average of six to eight colds a year, most of them between September and April.[7] This works out to about one a month. These colds last on average fourteen days.[8] A month is thirty days. So in the winter, on average, your kid will have a cold 50 percent of the time. On top of this, most kids end their cold with a cough that can last additional weeks. It adds up.

Most colds are minor, although they increase the risk of ear infection and other prolonged bacterial infections (bronchitis, walking pneumonia), which is why most doctors will tell you to come in if you are concerned, or if a fever lasts longer than a couple of days, or if your child gets worse after they've seemed to get better. Of these complications, ear infections are the most common. About a quarter of kids will have an ear infection by the age of one, and 60 percent by the age of four.[9]

If your kid does get sick, your doctor is your best resource. A very large share of sick visits to pediatricians are for colds, so although in many cases it's not necessary for your child to be seen by a doctor, you wouldn't be alone in having your kid checked out. You should also invest in a good general pediatrics book, which can do a more complete job at listing childhood symptoms than I can here. There are some references in the back; my favorite is *The Portable Pediatrician for Parents* by Laura Nathanson.

One thing that has changed since we were children: antibiotics. It used to be common to prescribe antibiotics for cold symptoms, at least some of the time. Not anymore.

Colds do not respond to antibiotics (they are caused by a virus), and your doctor shouldn't (and typically won't) prescribe them. Globally, overuse of antibiotics is a public health problem, since it contributes to antibiotic resistance. And even for your particular kid, antibiotics aren't totally risk-free—they can contribute to diarrhea, for example. The move toward prescribing antibiotics sparingly is definitely a good thing.

For ear infections or other complications, antibiotics may still be prescribed, although even for ear infections, they may not be necessary. The prescribing guidelines for this condition are complicated and depend a lot on what the ear looks like, along with other symptoms. If your kid's ear hurts, you are going to need to see your doctor.

In conclusion, enjoy your time in the land of snot! On the plus side, school-age kids get sick a bit less (two to four colds per year), so this doesn't last forever.

The Bottom Line

- Delayed motor development can be a signal of more serious issues, the most common of which is cerebral palsy.

- Variation in motor development within the (very wide) normal range is not a cause for concern.

- There are many approaches to evaluating motor skills; your pediatrician is your best partner in doing so.

- Children get many, many colds—about one per month for the winter, at least until school age. Lotion tissues. Lots of lotion tissues.

14

Baby Einstein vs.
the TV Habit

When I was a kid, we had one TV in the house. It was in the attic. My brothers and I were permitted to watch an hour of TV before dinner, and were limited to the PBS shows *3-2-1 Contact* and *Square One Television*. In seventh grade I finally convinced my mother to let me watch *90210*, since without it, I was doomed to social oblivion. I think she took pity on me in the hopes it would help (it didn't).

My parents' choice of programming—where *Square One* came after *Sesame Street*—reflected their desire to choose "educational" TV. Yes, we were allowed to watch TV, but at least it was something that would teach us letters and math.

Did we learn anything from these shows? I'm not sure. I certainly remember elements of *Square One* well—"Mathnet" and "Mathman" come to mind—but I do not associate them with any particular math concept. The one specific thing I do remember is a song—*You never reach infinity, you just go on . . . and on . . . .* I am sure I would have learned about infinity one way or another, but I think it is fair to credit the show. In the case of *Sesame Street*, there is actually good research suggesting that exposure to the show increases school readiness in kids ages three to five.

In the past thirty years, there has been tremendous progress both in educational programming and, in the past decade, other educational screen media. Where our parents had only *Sesame Street*, we as parents have a plethora of educational iPad games, DVDs, streaming videos, and so on. All of which promise early literacy and numeracy.

Sesame Street and similar shows (*Dora the Explorer, Blue's Clues*) are aimed largely at the preschool set. For younger children, the *Baby Einstein* DVDs reign. *Baby Einstein* is an enormously popular video franchise that produces content aimed at infants and toddlers with a combination of music, words, shapes, and pictures. The goal of these videos is explicitly educational. They aim to teach children new words, for example, or new music. And certainly the company claims they are successful.

On the other hand, there is a tremendous amount of evidence suggesting that exposure to TV—and, more generally, to any screens—is associated with lower cognitive development. Researchers have shown that kids who watch more TV are less healthy and have lower test scores.

Which is it? Is showing your nine-month-old a Baby Einstein DVD the way to encourage them to be an early talker? Or are you just developing the Berenstain Bears' dreaded "TV habit"?

The American Academy of Pediatrics falls squarely in agreement with the second answer. They recommend no TV or screen time at all for children under eighteen months, and no more than an hour a day, ideally consumed with a parent, for older children. In addition, they recommend choosing "high-quality" programming, such as that featured on PBS. That would include *Sesame Street*, although it would also include less learning-focused shows, such as the parent-despised Canadian-export *Caillou*.

But others argue that these recommendations are too conservative—and indeed, the AAP has wavered with them over time (until recently, it was no screen time until twenty-four months). The only way to answer is to go to the data.

BABY EINSTEIN

The field of developmental psychology is interested in—among other things—the question of how children learn. Researchers in this area bring kids, even young infants, into their labs and study how they interact with other people, with new toys, with different languages, and so on.

Within this research, we can start to learn about the potential for infants and toddlers to learn from videos. The results are not very encouraging. In one example, children twelve, fifteen, and eighteen months old were shown either a live person or a person on TV demonstrating some actions with puppets.[1] The researchers evaluated whether the children could repeat the action either in the moment or twenty-four hours later.

In all three age groups, when kids watched an actual person doing the action, some of them were able to replicate it a day later. The video demonstration was much less successful—the twelve-month-olds learned nothing, and the older kids learned much less than from seeing a live person do it.

Another example is a study where researchers tried to use a DVD recording to maintain exposure to non-native sounds. At birth, children are able to learn the sounds from any language, but as they age, they specialize in the sounds they hear regularly. Researchers tried to maintain exposure of English-speaking nine- to twelve-month-olds to Mandarin-language sounds, either through a live person or through a DVD.[2] The live person worked well, the DVD did not.[3]

These results suggest it would be surprising if Baby Einstein worked. But we can go further, since there is randomized trial evidence on this specific question.

In a 2009 paper, several researchers set out to test directly whether young children—in this case, twelve- to fifteen-month-olds—can learn words from DVDs.[4] They actually used a Baby Einstein product, a DVD called *Baby Wordsworth*, intended to increase vocabulary comprehension. Parents of children in the treatment group were given the DVD and told to have their children watch it regularly over six weeks. Children in the comparison group did not receive or watch the DVD.

Every two weeks, the researchers brought the children back into the lab and evaluated whether they had learned to either speak or understand new words. Over the course of the study, the number of words spoken and understood increased, since the kids aged. *However*, there were no differences in word learning in the DVD and non-DVD groups. The study's authors noted that the most significant predictor of both how many words the children spoke and how fast their vocabularies grew was whether their parents read them books. Other authors have extended versions of this study to kids up to age two and found similar results.[5]

Baby Einstein does not seem to live up to the name. This is not the way to bring your kid to the head of their day-care class. Of course, if you—*gasp!*—would like to use these videos to distract your kid while you, say, take a shower, vocabulary development may not be the goal. (More on the question of detrimental effects below.)

Videos may be a dud for baby learning. But there is more evidence that older kids can learn from television. If you have a preschooler and they watch any TV at all, you know this must be true. When Finn was two, he developed a disturbing habit of imitating Caillou ("But MOOOOMMM-MMYYYYY, I don't WAAANNNNTTTT to eat dinner"). He thought this was hilarious. There is no way he learned that from either us or his older sister.

Kids learn songs from movies and from shows, and can pick up names of characters and basic plot elements. Researchers in the lab have shown that three- to five-year-old kids are able to learn words from television.[6]

It shouldn't be surprising, then, that they can also pick up some good information. Perhaps the strongest evidence of this comes from studies of the show *Sesame Street*, which debuted in the 1970s to enormous popularity and wide acclaim. The goal of *Sesame Street* was explicitly learning based. The idea was to increase school readiness for kids ages three to five.

You can see this when you watch the show—they are focused on numbers, letters, and general pro-social behavior.

Early on, researchers used randomized trials to evaluate the effects of *Sesame Street*. In one evaluation, the group of families assigned to the treatment group had their televisions hooked up so they could access the show more effectively.[7] The researchers found, over a period of two years, improvements in various measures of school readiness, including vocabulary.

The effects of *Sesame Street* seem to be long-lived. A more recent study looked back at the early years of the show and compared the kids who got early access to it—because of better TV reception—to those who got later access. The earlier-access kids were less likely to be held back in school at older ages.[8] The show had bigger positive effects for children from more disadvantaged backgrounds, which could be due to differences in the other activities in their day, or to something else.

All this is to say that for slightly older children, television can be a source of some learning; this argues (among other things) for curation of what they watch. For very young children, what they watch may actually matter less, since they do not learn much from it, although you cannot rely on the TV to make your child a genius.

THE TV HABIT

Parental confession: I have never thought of television as a learning opportunity. My kids watch a bit of TV and it is heavily concentrated in time periods in which I need to get something done. At the end of the day on the weekend, when you've spent an entire day with the kids and need to cook dinner, it is awfully nice to send them off to watch TV for half an hour. The pull of the *Baby Einstein* videos for me was not that they would teach Finn anything, but that they might hold his attention for longer at a younger age.

If some quiet distraction is your goal, then your question is probably not whether TV is a learning opportunity, but whether it is detrimental. Does TV rot your child's brain?

Many studies say yes. For example, a 2014 study shows that preschoolers who watch more TV have lower "executive function"—meaning less self-control, focus, etc.[9] An earlier study, from 2001, shows obesity is higher among girls who watch more TV.[10]

These are just exemplars—many, many research papers correlate more television with bad outcomes. Among the most influential is a 2005 paper by Frederick Zimmerman and Dimitri Christakis.[11] Using a large, nationally representative dataset, their goal was to relate television watching at early ages to test scores among children ages six to seven. The researchers categorized the children into four groups based on how much TV they watched in two age ranges: under three years old, and three to five years old. "High" TV watching was more than three hours a day; "Low" was less than that.

Twenty percent of children fell into what they called the "High-High" group: more than three hours of TV a day both before age three and between ages three and five. Twenty-six percent fell into the "Low-High" group: less TV before age three, more from ages three to five. Fifty percent were in the "Low-Low" group, and just 5 percent fell into the "High-Low" group.

The authors reported the differences among the groups in math, reading, and vocabulary test scores at age six. Their results suggest that watching more TV under the age of three lowers test scores; not a huge amount, but by the equivalent of a couple of IQ points. If you are looking in this data for evidence that TV is bad, which is what the authors argue, high watching before age three seems to be an issue.

However, watching TV at older ages doesn't seem to matter. When the authors compared, say, the kids who watched only a little TV before age three and then a lot between ages three and five to the children who watched little TV before age three *and* little later, they found their test scores to be no different. If anything, the kids who watched more TV later had *higher* test scores than those who watched less.

This throws some cold water on the idea of avoiding TV for older children, but on its face, it does suggest that the recommendation of avoiding TV before age three is warranted. On the other hand, there are a few cautions. First, the kids in this study were watching a lot of TV. The average amount of television before the age of three is 2.2 hours *per day*, and the "High" TV group was watching more than 3 hours a day. It is challenging to extrapolate this to the question of, for example, whether you should allow your kid a couple of hours of TV per *week*.

Second, although the authors tried to control for this, it is very difficult to adjust for all the other differences between kids who watch a lot of TV and those who do not. The majority of the kids in the sample—75 percent— watched less TV between birth and age three; the ones who watched more must have been unusual in some ways. How do we know it was the TV and not these other things that matter? We can't, which is why this is a hard result to interpret.

Some researchers have tried to do a better job adjusting for this second issue, in particular. In my view, the best causal evidence on this comes from a 2008 paper by two economists, one of whom is my husband (but really! I think it is a good paper for other reasons!).[12] In fact, I like this paper so much that I also talked about it in *Expecting Better*. It's a good example of how to think about generating causal conclusions for a complicated question. It's also helpful for actual decisions about TV.

In the study, Jesse and his coauthor, Matt, took advantage of the fact that television was introduced to different areas of the United States at different times. This variation meant that when television was first introduced in the 1940s and '50s, some kids had access to TV when they were children and some did not. Since the timing of when people got TV in their area was not related to other parenting inputs, a lot of the concerns raised about other papers could be avoided.

The idea was to see how having TV access as a young child related to test scores when kids were in school at slightly older ages. Jesse and Matt found no evidence that more exposure to television at an early age negatively affected later test scores. This suggests the correlations in other data may be just that—correlations, not causal effects. Of course, TV in the 1940s and '50s differed from TV today, but kids in this time period did watch a lot of television, so the amount of TV isn't very different.

These studies all focus on TV. But in the current parenting climate, screen time has expanded. Your kid can now watch TV on your phone or iPad, but also play games and apps and do all manner of other things. Is this type of screen time like TV? Should it be limited?

We basically have no idea. There are a few studies, but they have pretty big flaws. An example is one paper—not even a paper, more of an abstract—that got a lot of press for showing that language delays were more common in children who had more exposure to a phone between the ages of six months and two years.[13] But this has the same problem, probably even more extreme, as the paper on TV discussed before. What other features of the family correlate with a lot of phone time for a six-month-old? Is it not possible that those features are what are associated with language delay?

This isn't to say that a lot of screen time is fine. We just do not really know.

LET'S BE BAYESIAN

The actual data we have on these questions is pretty limited. Based on what is available, I'd say we can learn a few things:

1. Children under two years old cannot learn much from TV.
2. Children ages three to five can learn from TV, including vocabulary and so on from programs like *Sesame Street*.
3. The best evidence suggests that TV watching in particular, even exposure at very young ages, does not affect test scores.

This may be helpful, but it leaves many questions unanswered. IPad apps—good or bad? Does sports on TV count as TV? Is there any amount of TV that's really *too* much? What about iPad shows—is the fact that there are no commercials a good thing or a bad thing?

Nothing in the data will answer these questions. But we can make more progress if we diversify our approach.

In the field of statistics, there are at least two broad approaches. The first is "frequentist statistics," which approaches learning about relationships in data using only the data we have. The second is "Bayesian statistics," which tries to learn about relationships by starting with a prior belief about the truth, and using data to update it.

To give an example in this context, let's say we have a well-run study that showed that kids who watch *SpongeBob SquarePants* are much more likely to be able to read at the age of two, and that this is the only study on this topic. In the world of frequentist statistics, you'd be forced to conclude that *SpongeBob* is a great learning tool.

For a Bayesian, this conclusion is less clear. Before seeing the data, we are very unlikely to think that *SpongeBob* can teach two-year-olds to read. Observing the data should make us more likely to think this relationship is real, but if we start out very skeptical, we should remain quite skeptical even after seeing the data.

A Bayesian approach is to think about how to incorporate other things you know—or think you know—about the world into your conclusion along with the data.

Why is this relevant here? I think we have some prior beliefs on this topic. There are only thirteen or so waking hours in the day for kids. If they spend eight of those hours watching TV, there is not enough time to do pretty much anything else. It seems very unlikely that this won't have some negative impacts.

On the other hand, it is hard to imagine that watching an hour a week of *Sesame Street* or *Dora the Explorer* will lower your child's IQ, or have much of any effect on them in the long run.

You can subject the iPad to similar logic. A two-year-old who is on an iPad all day: likely bad. A half hour of math games twice a week: probably not bad.

When we start from this point, the data—while sparse—looks a lot more helpful, since it actually provides a lot of information about precisely the things we have less intuition about (what's known in the Bayesian approach as "having a weaker prior").

For example, I don't have much intuition about whether young children can learn from videos. The data—which indicates they cannot—is therefore very informative and useful. Similarly, although I have a good sense that watching eight hours of TV a day is bad and an hour a week is fine, I have less intuition about "normal" watching—in the realm of, say, two hours per day. For this question, Jesse's work is quite informative, since it looks at precisely this magnitude of exposure and shows there is no impact.

If I want to map out the whole relationship between test scores and any amount of TV, I am still not done, but I can start to use the combination of my priors—my beliefs before I saw the data—and what we do see from the data to fill in where I was most uncertain.

This starts to give us a sense, as well, of where more studies might be most useful. Many kids use apps on iPads or tablets for some time every day. We basically have no research on this, and it's not something about which one is likely to have very good intuition. I could believe that this is good—there are many very neat apps for math and reading. I could also believe it is bad—you're not really *learning*, you're just tapping around.

Finally, our intuitions should be informed by the economic idea of "opportunity cost of time." If a child is watching TV, they are not doing something else. Depending on what that "something else" is, TV watching may be better or worse. Many studies of this emphasize that (for example) your kid can learn letters or vocabulary from *Sesame Street*, but they are better at learning those things from you. That's almost certainly true, but it is less obvious to me that this is the alternative. Many parents use TV to take a break, get their breath, make a meal, do some laundry. If the alternative to an hour of TV is a frantic and unhappy parent yelling at their kid for an hour, there is good reason to think the TV might actually be better.

The Bottom Line

- Your zero- to two-year-old cannot learn from TV.
- A three- to five-year-old can learn from TV.
  - It is worth paying attention to what they are watching.
- The evidence is sparse overall. When in doubt, use your "Bayesian priors" to complement the data.

15

Slow Talking, Fast Talking:
Language Development

When I was twenty-two months old, my parents (both also economists—I know, I know) were at a cocktail party, and my mother struck up a conversation with a visiting professor, Katherine Nelson. Her field was child language development, and my mother mentioned that she had a daughter (me) who talked a lot, especially alone in her crib prior to falling asleep. Professor Nelson got very excited and asked if my mother would be willing to consider recording my crib speech, for research. Indeed, she would.

For the next eighteen months or so, my parents recorded me most nights and provided the tapes to Professor Nelson and her team of researchers. Early on, my mother transcribed many of the tapes to try to make sense of my poor diction. This large corpus of tapes and text—some of it of me talking alone, some talking with my parents—provided a trove of data for researchers studying how children acquire language. They were interested in questions like, does the concept of the future develop for kids before the concept of the past? There were papers, academic conferences, and eventually a book of collected research papers on the tapes.

(The irony of both being the subject of a book like this and also writing one is not lost on me.)

This book—*Narratives from the Crib*[1]—came out when I was about nine. I have a vivid memory of coming home from school and finding an advance copy on the table in the porch. I opened it, eager for some insights into my younger self, but sadly found it somewhat lacking in that department. This was a dry academic book—a set of papers written by linguists analyzing verb form and sentence structure. I remember reading some of the funnier quotes from me and putting it aside.

I didn't really look at the book again until Penelope was getting to the same age. And this time it was in service of the perennial parental neurosis: comparing your child to others. I scoured the book to try to figure out how Penelope and I compared. The earliest quote in the book is, "When Daddy comes I put that there then eat my breakfast and Daddy make my bed," from twenty-two months and five days. Was Penelope saying things like that at a similar age? It was hard to tell—I pushed my mother: "Did I really say that, or was that just what you thought I said?" Needless to say, she could not remember. (Or so she claimed.)

Communicating with one another—talking, signing, writing—is among the things that make us most human. The moment your child stops having to cry and point desperately at the refrigerator and can instead say, "Milk, please" (or even just "MILK!!") is one in which you can start to see glimmers of a person in there. We usually remember our children's first words (Penelope: "shoes"; Finn: "Penelope [Puh-Puh]"), and early on many of us will probably admit to counting just how many they have.

Talking is also a natural point of comparison—of your children to other children, of your children to each other, and (in my case) of your children to yourself. I was warned before I had Finn that this problem is especially acute if you have a daughter first, followed by a son.

"Boys are slower with language," warned my more delicate friends. Some less delicate ones said, "You'll think your son is stupid." People whose children were born in the opposite gender order told me how brilliant they thought their daughter was.

Figuring out how your child compares with others is not, in fact, straight-forward. As with physical milestones, doctors tend to focus on identifying children for early intervention. At the two-year-old doctor visit, it is common to be asked whether the child has at least twenty-five words they say regularly. At fewer than this, it may be appropriate to bring in some outside help to figure out what is wrong. But this is a cutoff to indicate a problem, not a measure of the average or anything about the range. The average child has more than twenty-five words at age two. But how *many* more?

Most pediatrics books have similar approaches—they warn you when to be concerned, but don't give a sense of the full distribution.

Even with the full distribution, there are other questions: Does it matter? Is talking early a marker of anything later? Both of these questions have answers—the first a bit more satisfying than the second—we just have to go to the data.

THE DISTRIBUTION OF WORDS

In principle, it seems like it would be straightforward to collect data on how many words children say. Specifically, you could just count them. And it's true that when a child is very small—when they have five or ten or twenty words—probably parents could remember most of them if asked. But this procedure can break down as children talk more and more. Let's say your child says four hundred words, some of them used frequently and some infrequently. Will you really remember them all?

A related problem in comparisons is how to count words that are specific to your child. For example: At just over two, Finn became obsessed with a song entitled "Bumblebee Variety Show," written by the local Music To-gether instructor, Jen. We played it on repeat every time we were in the car. He liked to sing it loudly—in the car with the music, in his crib, in the bath.

The primary lyrics in this song are "Bumblebee variety show." Techni-cally, then, he could say this, although he pronounced it as one word:

bumblebeevarietyshow. So: When counting words, should I think of him as knowing the word *variety*? He certainly would not use it in a sentence, nor did he think of it as a separate word. So, probably not. But then should I count *bumblebeevarietyshow* as a single word? This seems more plausible. But still, it's not even clear he thought of this as a word as opposed to just a noise. Also, it is actually *not* a word.

Researchers get around both of these problems—recall and the comparison set—by using a standardized measure of vocabulary size from a consistently used survey. The commonly used one is the MacArthur-Bates Communicative Development Inventory (MB-CDI).

The MB-CDI is administered to parents (Want to do it yourself? See the endnotes).[2] The vocabulary portion lists 680 words in various categories—animal sounds, action words (*bite*, *cry*), body parts, etc. Parents check off all the words they have heard their child say, giving them a count of vocabulary size on these words.

For kids above sixteen months, the survey uses words and sentences; for those younger than that, there is a separate form for words and gestures.

This approach to vocabulary size works well for two reasons. First, by listing the words and asking about them rather than asking parents to remember, parents are less likely to forget words. I may not be able to recall without prompting that my son knew the word *shovel*, but once it is mentioned, I may remember an incident in which he asked for one. Second, by looking at the same words for every kid, it is much easier to compare across children.

An obvious downside to this approach is that it will understate speaking ability for children who know a lot of unusual words but miss some common ones. For example, one of the words on the list is *Coke*; if your children do not drink soda, they may not know this word. Similarly, children in Hawaii may be less familiar with the word *sled*.

This problem is most acute as you get to ages where children know most of the words. It may not really be feasible to distinguish between a child who says 675 of the words and one who says 680. For children who know fewer words, these small differences balance out—one child knows *sled*, another knows *beach*.

Many people have completed this form. Much of this is in service of research. Some is in service of evaluating children for developmental delays or simply to satisfy curious parents. Regardless of the reason, the developers of this survey have a website where results can be uploaded. And from this, we can get a first answer to the question of the distribution of words. The graph below was created out of their data—the horizontal axis is the age, and the vertical axis is the count of words as scored in the survey.

The lines in the graph show "quantiles"—basically, the distribution of words at each age. Take, for example, age 24 months. This data says that the average child—that's the 50th percentile line—at 24 months has about 300 words. A child at the 10th percentile—so, near the bottom of the distribution—has only about 75 words. On the other end, a child at the 90th percentile has close to 550 words.

For younger children, these surveys and data focus on both words and gestures (i.e., signs). The graph on page 233 shows similar data for children

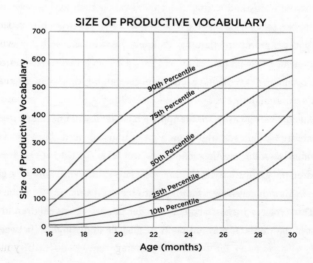

SIZE OF PRODUCTIVE VOCABULARY

aged eight to eighteen months on this metric. One main takeaway from these graphs is the explosion of language after fourteen or sixteen months. Even the most advanced one-year-old has only a few words. At eight months, virtually no children have any words or gestures.

I was interested to note this, given my mother-in-law's continual insistence that Jesse said the word *fishy* at six months.

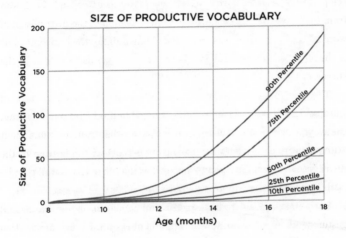

SIZE OF PRODUCTIVE VOCABULARY

The website for this data is publicly accessible[3] and has the capacity to make all sorts of graphs—they can show you the data broken down by parental education or birth order (later children talk more slowly), for example, and they have similar data for other languages and for counts of words children understand in addition to being able to speak. It is worth noting here that kids who are bilingual—that is, their parents or caregivers speak to them in two different languages—tend to be slower to talk, although when they do, they can speak both languages.

Perhaps the most interesting of these splits is by gender, given the general impression that boys develop more slowly. This is, indeed, borne out in the data. The graphs on page 234 separate out boys and girls, and we can see that boys have fewer words at all points in the distribution. At twenty-four months, for example, the average girl has about fifty more words than the average boy. By thirty months, the most advanced boys and girls are similar, but there are still large differences at other points in the distribution.

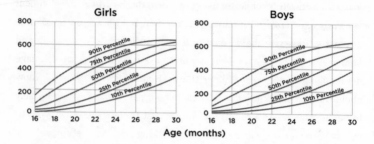

This data provides some useful norming, but it is important to be cautious about where it comes from. It is not (for the most part) nationally representative data. There are many more parents with college or graduate degrees in these data points than you would see in the overall population. This means these figures are likely to overstate the average among all children. Having said that, they give you something beyond a general guideline about when to be worried, and also provide reassurance that there is a significant range in this distribution at all young ages.

DOES IT MATTER ANYWAY?

We all enjoy navel-gazing about our own children, so knowing where your child falls in this distribution may be simply a fun fact. But virtually everyone learns to talk. It is natural to wonder, though, whether these early differences do predict any long-term differences. Do children who learn to talk earlier learn to read earlier? Do they do better in school later?

There are certainly counterexamples to this idea—stories of extremely precocious children who didn't talk until very late but were reading at eighteen months. And there are also supportive stories: early talkers who also turned out to be unusual in other ways. But examples like this, in either direction, do not tell us anything about the relationship on average.

To echo a refrain from throughout this book, this is difficult to learn about given other relationships in the data. Language development is clearly associated with parental education. But parental education is also associated with many other outcomes, including early reading and later test scores. What we'd really like to ask is whether early language development is a marker of later things, *conditional* on what we know about the parents. But our information about parents in the data is likely to be incomplete. As a result, the studies that I'll talk about are likely to overstate the relationship between early talking and later outcomes.

There are basically two questions you could ask here: Can you take anything from your child being either a very strong early talker or a very delayed one? And, assuming your child is in the middle of the distribution, does it matter where they are? Are there any later-life differences between a two-year-old who is at the 25th percentile of the distribution versus the 50th, or the 75th?

The largest and most rigorous studies of this focus on whether children who are abnormally late talkers are also delayed in other ways later.

In a series of studies, a researcher named Leslie Rescorla recruited a set of thirty-two delayed talkers from twenty-four to thirty-one months old.[4] The children in this delayed cohort—nearly all boys—had an average of twenty-one words at this age. Based on the previous graphs, this is way below average. She recruited a sample of comparison children with similar characteristics but with normally developing language skills.

Notably, this study followed the children—or at least most of them—to much later ages, up to age seventeen. At older ages, researchers looked at verbal abilities, test scores, and similar outcomes.[5]

The results provide a mixed bag of evidence. On one hand, the group with delays in talking did seem to have slightly worse outcomes on the tests even much later. Their IQ scores at age seventeen were lower than the comparison group. On the other hand, these children were not especially likely to score very poorly—none of them scored in the bottom 10 percent on IQ tests at seventeen, for example, despite having been in the bottom 10 percent of talkers.

This basic result—that there is a correlation, but the predictive power is limited—is consistent across many studies. Some of the studies are much bigger. For example, a paper reporting on six thousand children in the Early Childhood Longitudinal Study found that limited vocabulary at twenty-four months predicts verbal skills through the age of five, but again, most of the children were well in the normal ranges later.[6]

These studies focus on delayed talkers. Within the normal range, we have less work, but there is at least one 2011 paper entitled "Size Matters" (I guess it's funny?) that compares children who are earlier versus later talkers at the age of two.[7] Their "later-talking" group had an average of 230 words at age two, versus 460 for the high talkers. These are different portions of the distribution, but in the normal range.

Studying kids through age eleven, this paper again found lasting differences across the groups, but there was a lot of overlap. To give a sense of this: On one measure of language ability (something called "word attack") at grade 1, the later-talking group had an average score of 104, versus 110 in the early-talking group. Clearly, the early-talking group was doing better. But there was also a huge amount of variation within each group.

The following graph gives a sense of the range for the two groups.[8] On one hand, we can see the (on average) higher scores in the early-talking group. On the other hand, there is a tremendous amount of overlap in the distributions. The individual variation completely swamps the difference in averages.

What about really exceptional language ability? Again, we see some small-scale evidence that being a precocious talker correlates with precocity later.[9] But this correlation is not enormous in this or other studies, and being a very good talker before two is by no means a decisive determinant of early reading or other achievements.[10]

It is natural, probably unavoidable, for us as parents to want to compare our children to others. Language development is among the first

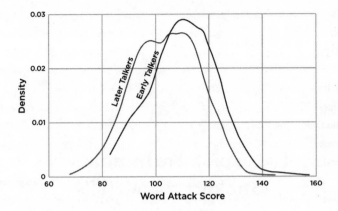

cognitive processes that we really see in kids, so it is not surprising that it becomes a focus of comparison. And if you are really curious, it's definitely possible to use the data here to do some more concrete comparisons. But it is crucial to keep in mind that the predictive ability of early language, while there, is really quite poor. Early talking doesn't guarantee later success—even at four—and late talkers mostly look like everyone else within a few years.

The Bottom Line

- There are some standard tools to determine child vocabulary size, which you can use on your own. There are also some metrics you can compare.
- Girls develop language faster than boys, on average, although there is a lot of overlap across genders.
- The timing of language development does have some link with later outcomes—test scores, reading—but the predictive power is weak for any individual child.

Potty Training:
Stickers vs. M&M's

My mother is fond of telling the story of how I was potty trained. "When you were twenty-two months old, one day you announced you would now be using big-girl underwear. That was a Friday, and on Monday, I brought you back to day care without diapers."

This story is implausible on several levels (the announcement, the speed of training, and so on). When she first told me this, I also thought the age was impossible. Twenty-two months? I think not. And it is true that usually when we return to her written notes on topics like this (yes, I know that not everyone's mother kept detailed written notes—it's a family affair), she is often revealed to have exaggerated. However, in this case, she did not. Her notes from the time suggest, largely without comment, that I was wearing underwear by this age.

Not to be outdone, my mother-in-law insists Jesse was potty trained by eighteen months, and pooped in the toilet at thirteen months. She also suggests this was pretty typical.

But I distinctly remember that my younger brother (sorry, Steve) was not potty trained when he started preschool at age three. This was unusual at the time, and was a source of a tremendous amount of parental anxiety.

The question of when to potty train remains a source of stress for parents. Should you push your child to train early? If you do, will you stress them out? If you don't, will they be somehow behind?

And the experience of our parents' generation, and therefore of the grandparents who are speaking over our shoulders, doesn't seem necessarily typical now. My brother, a late potty trainer by the standards of the time, seems like he would be quite typical now. Training at eighteen months—especially for a boy—sounds like the more unusual thing.

This is, however, only my casual impression, and I was curious if it lined up with any actual data. I decided to be a bit more systematic. In other words, rather than just asking my friends, I ran a survey. I sent it to my friends, their parents, their parents' friends, people on Facebook and Twitter—basically anyone I could find. I asked a few simple questions: When was your child born? And when were they potty trained?

The first graph on page 240 shows the average age of potty training by birth timing in my survey.[1] And, indeed, the average age has crept up over time—from thirty months for births before 1990 to more than thirty-two months in the most recent period. But perhaps even more notable is the second graph, which shows the share of children who are trained at or after thirty-six months (that's three years). This was only about 25 percent of the children in the earliest birth years, but 35 to 40 percent in the most recent period.

Of course, this is not exactly a scientifically valid sample. It definitely would not pass peer review. But the casual impression—and the findings from this data—is supported by the literature. Studies from the 1960s and '80s show an average age of twenty-five to twenty-nine months for daytime toilet-training completion, and virtually all the children were trained (for the daytime) by thirty-six months. In contrast, in more recent cohorts only 40 to 60 percent of children have trained by thirty-six months.[2]

This suggests toilet training is occurring later. Why?

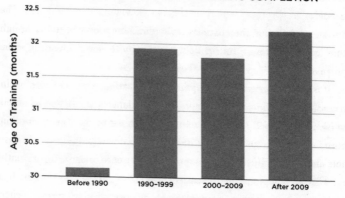

AVERAGE AGE OF POTTY TRAINING COMPLETION

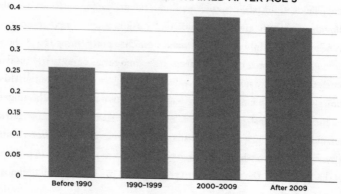

SHARE OF CHILDREN TRAINED AFTER AGE 3

The *Journal of Pediatrics* published a study in 2004 asking this very question.[3] The study enrolled four hundred children when they were about eighteen months old and followed them through potty training. They found three factors significantly associated with later training. The first—and probably the one that explains variation over time—is later initiation of potty training. Children who start training later complete training later.

The other two factors relate to poop. Children who were frequently constipated, or who showed resistance to pooping in the potty (formally "stool toileting refusal"—more on this to follow) tended to train later. The authors argued that these factors could also increase over time, although they largely put the blame for later training on the later initiation of the process.

It is interesting to speculate why people have started training later in recent years. My mother insists it relates to diaper quality—diapers used to leak a lot, which made it much less fun to use them. The generation born in the late 1970s and early '80s was the first to commonly use disposable diapers, perhaps due to innovations in the early 1980s that dramatically decreased the size of disposable diapers.[4]

Income may also play a role. People have become, on average, richer over time, and the inflation-adjusted price of diapers has gone down. This may make a prolonged period of diaper wearing more acceptable, although affording diapers is still a challenge for many families.

There is likely also some feedback loop. If everyone potty trains their child when they turn two, people may feel some social pressure in this direction. If everyone else waits until three, that becomes the norm. This may also affect when, for example, day-care centers push potty training.

Regardless of why this occurs, the fact that later initiation correlates with later completion suggests that it is, in fact, possible to potty train your kid at a younger age. Should you do so?

The main and probably only benefit to potty training a child earlier is that you do not have to change as many diapers. The main reason to wait is that the earlier you start, the longer it takes to complete. We can see this in the same data described above, with the 400 children starting at 18 months.

The first graph on page 242, re-created from their study,[5] shows the age of completion of potty training as a function of the age of initiation (both of these are as reported by the parents). Here they define the age of initiation as the first age at which parents *try* to train their kid—as in, asking the child at least three times a day if they need to use the potty. And the age of completion is when the parents say the kid is fully trained in the daytime.

What we can see is that the age of potty-training completion is similar starting anytime between twenty-one and thirty months. The second graph shows the duration of potty training—the earlier you start, the longer it takes to complete. A somewhat depressing aspect of this graph is that the duration of training is about a year if you start young.

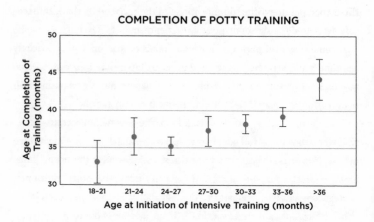

COMPLETION OF POTTY TRAINING

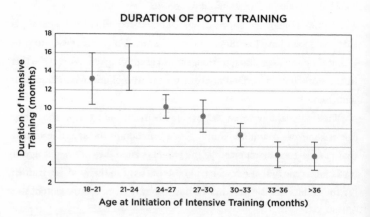

DURATION OF POTTY TRAINING

The authors suggest that if what you care about is when potty training is done, there is not much point to starting before twenty-seven months or so. But it is the case that after this, starting earlier does generally mean finishing earlier. If you start training at twenty-seven or twenty-eight months, you can expect to be done by around age three, but it will take ten months to do it. If you start at age three, you finish later, but it'll likely take you less than six months to fully train.

As we think about the contrast between doing this at age two and doing it at three, it is worth thinking about the ways in which your two- and three-year-old are different that makes this harder or easier. A three-year-old has a lot more control over their bathroom functions (also maybe over you, but that is a different story). This is partly physical, and partly emotional. An eighteen-month-old is much less likely to simply decide they will not poop in the potty no matter what you say. They have less will to defy you. This may make littler kids easier.

On the other hand, a three-year-old can be reasoned with and—yes—bribed. They have more will to defy you, but you can also take advantage of their better ability to understand and control themselves. That may make them easier to deal with. The data on timing suggests that, on net, the latter probably matters more.

METHODS

Having chosen a time to start your potty-training adventure, there is then the question of how to do it. Broadly, potty-training approaches come in one of two forms.

First, there is the parent-led, "endpoint-oriented" potty training.[6] These methods are discussed in books like *Oh Crap!* and *3-Day Potty Training*. In general, the idea is to just take the diapers away and start putting your child on the potty a lot. Ideally, within a few days they are (mostly) trained. There are less intense (and more intense) versions of this as well, but they all share the same basic structure: parents decide when it is time to potty train and then push toward the end goal. Based on the timing data we saw earlier, either most people do not use these approaches or most people do not use them successfully.

(I have promised my children that I will not discuss their potty-training adventures in detail here, but I will say that we did use this method, and broadly I was happy with it. However, it worked better for one child than the other, and we definitely did not achieve full success in three days.)

On the other side is a more laissez-faire approach, where you more or less let the child lead with the timing that works for them. This approach involves looking for signs of readiness and encouraging toilet use when they become apparent. This is goal oriented in the sense that ultimately you would like the child to use the toilet, but it does not work on the same time frame.

There is a third approach, "Elimination Communication," which tries to have kids use the potty from birth. More on this in a bit.

These approaches were developed many years ago—the original description of child-led potty training is from 1962. A major difference between them is the age at which they seem plausible—generally, using a child-led approach will involve starting later.

There is virtually no data on which of these works better or even how well any individual system works.[7] To the extent there are studies on this, they are extremely difficult to interpret. Consider, for example, one study of twenty children (twenty!), which considered a potty-training intervention in a preschool classroom.[8] The program contained three different interventions (using underwear, making the child sit on the potty frequently, and rewarding potty use). With a subset of the children, researchers had the preschool teachers do all three. With others, they did them sequentially.

Some children improved, some did not. There were virtually no consistent associations. The best the study authors could say was that many of the children who wore underwear seemed to improve. And, perhaps most important, that all the children were eventually toilet trained.

There are other small studies. One, of thirty-nine children in the UK, compared a wetting alarm method (where children are fitted with a special diaper that plays an alarm when they pee in the diaper) with a method of putting the child on the potty at regular intervals. They found evidence that the wetting alarm was more effective, but again, this was a small sample and not a comprehensive study of particular approach. Also, clearly the alarm approach won't be for everyone.

If you are desperate for some evidence-based guidance, one randomized study of seventy-one children from 1977 compared a child-led approach to an intensive one.[9] The study argues in support of the more intensive method, showing that accidents per day declined more in the intensive training group, and successes went up more. But this study is very old and small, and didn't look at any other outcomes for the children (for example, were they stressed out about the training).

The main thrust of the literature on this is that we simply do not know much about the best methods, if there even is a single best method.

This last point is probably the most important: there may not be a single best method for every child or every family.

When my twin nephews were being potty trained, my mother made a book to read to them, entitled *The Lion Gets Potty Trained*. It featured a series of pictures of my niece (their older sister) and a stuffed lion. The theme is that she was attempting to train the lion to use the toilet using various rewards—M&M's, Skittles, a kumquat, etc. Finally, she is successful by offering the lion a meatball.

I have read this book to Finn many times, and in many ways it really epitomizes this experience. You will try anything—literally anything!—to get your child to use the bathroom, but you cannot actually force them. And, probably most important, all kids are different. Some kids respond to stickers. Some respond to M&M's. Maybe some respond to meatballs.

The bottom line is that potty training is really all about what works for your family and your kid. The evidence on changes over time suggests it is possible to train your child at a younger age than is now typical, if you want to. To do this, you'll probably have to adopt a more goal-oriented approach (rather than a child-led approach). Or you can wait until your child decides they are ready, which will probably be when they are closer to three years old or even a bit older.

The child-led approach to training may take longer, but it also may be more pleasant for you. Or maybe this is your last child, you are totally over changing diapers, and you want your twenty-five-month-old to get with the program. If this is the case, your best bet is probably to try an intensive, goal-oriented regime and see if she takes to it.

There is no evidence linking age of potty training with any later outcomes like IQ or education.[10] So if your child is trained early, that might be great (for you) but irrelevant in the long term. It may be hard to see through the haze of running your child to the bathroom every twenty minutes and cleaning up the poop in their underwear, but everyone does eventually use the toilet.

PROBLEMS AND EXTENSIONS

Stool Toileting Refusal

At some point, before Penelope was born, I had a conversation with a friend about her son. How are things going? I asked her. "He's doing well, although of course we are dealing with an STR issue."

"A what?"

"Oh, stool toileting refusal."

This was my first exposure (but not the last) to the seemingly widespread "STR" problem, which I continue to feel is a great name for your child not pooping in the toilet.

This problem is surprisingly common (or, rather, surprising for people who do not have children yet). Perhaps a quarter of kids will experience some degree of this during potty training.[11] As weird as it might sound, a lot of kids like to poop in their diaper. Children who will successfully urinate in the toilet will nevertheless refuse to poop there, and unlike urine, bowel movements are something over which even young children do have some control.

When the refusal to have a bowel movement in the toilet continues well past when kids regularly urinate in the toilet, this rises to the level of a problem. The main issue is that withholding poop can cause constipation. This can lead to painful bowel movements when they finally arrive, which further exacerbates the problem. Now the child associates using the toilet with pain and *really* doesn't want to do it. Chronic constipation can also lead to problems with urination.

There is some work studying how to address this issue in older children—stool withholding is also a common issue in school-age children—but virtually nothing systematic in younger ages.[12] One study of four hundred children, published in 2003, showed that the length of refusal (i.e., the number of months this goes on) decreased with a child-oriented intervention where, among other things, parents made a big deal about the child pooping in the diaper before potty training started.[13] This means saying things like, "Wow! You pooped! That's so great!" and so on. The kids in this treatment were no less likely to have the problem at all, but it lasted for less time.

A common piece of advice to address this issue is that the child be given a diaper to poop in, perhaps in the bathroom. Although it may seem like a step backward, the theory is that it lowers the chance of constipation and subsequent negative feedback. There is not much evidence on this in either direction. In at least one small prospective study, children who were put back in diapers were virtually all trained within three months. But again, with time, everyone uses the toilet, and without a control group, it is difficult to learn much.[14]

Nighttime Dryness

Staying dry at night—or effectively waking up to use the bathroom—is a skill fundamentally different from using the toilet during the day. Many children will remain in a pull-up or diaper at night (and maybe when napping) long after they are fully trained during the day.

In contrast to the day, staying dry at night basically requires that your body wakes you up if and when you need to pee. This ability develops at different ages in different children. By the age of five, 80 to 85 percent of children are dry at night (meaning not that they do not pee, but that if they do, they wake to use the bathroom).[15]

Doctors generally do not worry about lack of nighttime dryness until a child is six years old. Older than that, it is common to begin to consider some interventions—waking the child to pee, limiting fluids before bed, a wetting alarm. These continued issues affect perhaps 10 percent of children (mostly boys) and nearly all of them eventually resolve.

ELIMINATION COMMUNICATION

Most people take for granted that their child will spend some time in diapers. Elimination communication, however, is a method in which parents train—perhaps from birth—to recognize the signs that their child is going to pee or poop and then quickly put them on the potty. Obviously with a baby that cannot sit up yet, you cannot put them on a toilet—the idea here is to hold them in your lap over a bowl or similar so they get the association.

There are very few studies about elimination communication. One early report surveyed parents engaging this strategy and showed that, indeed, many parents reported their child did give signs of needing to use the toilet, even at a very young age.[16] The children in the study were trained very early—by seventeen months, on average—with no adverse effects.

It is worth noting that elimination communication is billed not as an explicit potty-training method, but as a system designed to encourage toilet use. It is hard to know what is meant by this distinction, but I think it is that in doing formal "potty training," you are aiming to accomplish your goal in a relatively short time, whereas starting at infancy means this will necessarily take more time.

Other studies are anecdotal reports of success, or summary articles that note that in cultures without diapers, moms seem to learn earlier how to figure out a child is about to go.

If you think this is appealing, there is no reason not to do it, although it is probably worth noting that it is a reasonably impactful lifestyle choice and not one you are likely to get much support on from, say, your day care.

The Bottom Line

- Age at toilet training has increased over time, very likely as a result of parents choosing to train later.

- Starting training earlier leads to earlier completion on average, although it generally takes longer; starting intensive training before twenty-seven months does not seem to lead to earlier completion.

- There is little evidence on the efficacy of child-led training versus more intensive, goal-oriented methods.

- Refusal to poop on the toilet is a common complication with some limited solutions.

Toddler Discipline

When I misbehaved as a small child, my mother's solution was to ask me to "sit on the stairs and think about it." I would toddle off to the stairs, sit for a while and contemplate my wrongs, and then return to explain what I did wrong and that I would not do it again. My mother congratulated herself on being an amazing parent who was deeply in touch with her child and didn't need to resort to the kind of "Go to your room!" discipline that others practiced.

Then my brother, Stephen, arrived.

He did not want to sit on the stairs and think about it when he misbehaved. In fact, he loudly refused. Things escalated to his being sent to his room. Also refused. My mother found herself physically carrying him to his room, shutting the door, and holding the door closed with all her strength while he screamed and tried to get out.

Which goes to show, again, that parenting is much more about the child than about the parent. (Sidenote: Stephen is a wonderful and successful adult who was and remains a great brother.)

When my own kids were born, I repeated a similar pattern. Penelope never had a tantrum. When Finn had one, I couldn't believe it. There was so much yelling! I asked Jesse, "Do you think he's sick? Should we take him to the doctor?" Jesse looked at me like I was a crazy person. "He's not sick. He's two."

Tantrums are at the more extreme end of toddler acting out, and nearly everyone has a story about one, usually one that occurred in public. When I talked to my friend Jenna about this chapter, she said her mom is still angry about a tantrum Jenna had at age four in a Kmart. My nephew once had one in a crowded mall, leaving his mother to walk away (the correct response) while he screamed on the floor and people stopped to try to help. Of course, once a child is in a tantrum, there is really no helping.

Toddlers act out in other ways as well. They can almost seem like scientists—experimenting with what is possible. *If I throw this half-eaten cauliflower stem at Mom and say, "I don't LIKE IT!," what will happen? If I hit my sister on the head with a book, will she hit back? Will an adult stop me?*

The constant experimentation can be exhausting and confusing, especially as your kid gets to the point where it is harder to physically restrain them. When your son insists on repeatedly taking his shirt off in a museum, what do you do? Do you physically put the shirt back on? Do you just give up and let him run around without a shirt? (Why does he want to take the shirt off anyway? He repeatedly emphasized his intense desire to wear that very shirt in the morning.)

The somewhat good news is that there are evidence-based approaches to dealing with discipline. I say "somewhat good" since there is no magic bullet that will completely stop tantrums and turn your two-year-old into a seven-year-old. Instead, parenting interventions focus on how to respond to bad behavior when it starts and limit recurrence.

Before even getting into evidence, though, it's worth stepping back and thinking about why we want to discipline our kids. What are we trying to accomplish? I think the answer is the same as what we are trying to do with all our other parenting choices: we are trying to raise happy, nice, productive adults. When my kid refuses to clean up a mess and I discipline that behavior, it is not really that I want some help cleaning up. Actually, it would be faster to clean up myself than get her to do it. It's more that I'm trying to teach her to be someone who takes responsibility for her messes, both the LEGO messes now and the inevitable non-LEGO messes she'll create in the future.

This is the discipline-as-education philosophy espoused by French parenting (thanks, *Bringing Up Bébé!*). Discipline is not the same as punishment. Yes, there is a punishment component. But it's in the service of raising better humans, not punishment for its own sake.

With this scaffolding, we can turn to the data. There are a number of evidence-based parenting interventions. These include 1-2-3 Magic, the Incredible Years, Triple P—Positive Parenting Program, and so on. Many schools—including those that have children with serious behavioral issues—use a similar program called Positive Behavior Interventions and Supports, which has a similar set of goals and structures.

Broadly, all these emphasize a few key elements.

First, recognize that children are not adults, and you usually cannot improve their behavior with a discussion. If your four-year-old is taking their shirt off in the museum, they will not respond to a reasoned discussion about how you actually do need to wear a shirt in public places. The flip side of this—more important—is that you shouldn't expect them to respond to adult reasoning. And as a result, you should not get angry the way you would if, say, your spouse was stripping in the museum and didn't stop after you explained why they shouldn't.

All these interventions emphasize not getting angry. Don't yell, don't escalate, and definitely don't hit. Controlling parental anger is the first central part of the intervention.

This is so easy to say, but it is often *so hard to do*. It takes practice on your part. Most of us do not want to get angry with our kids, but we have all found ourselves furious in various moments. Toddler discipline is, really, parental discipline. Breathe. Take a second. I once told my children,

"I'm so mad right now, I'm going to the bathroom for a while to calm down." (It's the only door in the house that locks.) And I did, only coming out when I thought I could handle not only them, but myself.

An extension of this your-child-is-not-an-adult observation is that it is probably not a good use of your time to think a lot about why your small child is having a tantrum. There is a strong temptation to try to figure out what exactly is the issue—to try to get them to articulate the precise problems they are having. Even if they can talk, this is likely to be fruitless, since they probably do not know. Tantrums happen for all kinds of reasons. Working on disciplining the tantrum behavior is the goal. If they do not think of a tantrum as a way to react, they can work on developing other, more productive ways to communicate their problems.

Second, these approaches all emphasize setting up a clear system of rewards and punishments and following through on them every time. For example, 1-2-3 Magic develops a system of counting (to three, obviously) in the face of disruptive behavior, and if three is reached, there is a defined consequence (a time-out, loss of a privilege, etc.).

Finally, there is a strong emphasis on consistency. Whatever the system you use, use it every time. If the consequence of counting to three is a time-out, then there needs to be a time-out *every time*, including, say, in the grocery store. (The book suggests you find a corner of the store, or bring a "time-out mat" with you.)

As an extension, if you say no to something, you stick to no. If your kid asks for dessert and you say no, you cannot then later say yes if they whine for long enough. This basically makes sense—what do they learn from that? That whining will sometimes work. Let's do more of it! And similarly, do not make threats you cannot carry out.

Let's say you are on an airplane and your child keeps kicking the seat in front of them. Telling them, "If you do that one more time, I'm going to leave you on the airplane" is not a good threat. Why? Because you are not going to leave them on the airplane. When they then kick again to test this, and they find they are not, in fact, left on the airplane, they'll file this away for later. The same logic goes for the common parent car trip threat, "I'm going to turn this car around if you kids do not stop fighting!" Fine to say this, but you'd better be prepared to turn around.

These are the broad parameters. Like sleep training, the specifics differ across programs. If you are hoping to use this kind of discipline, you'll probably want to pick a particular program and stick to it. One may not be better than the other, but given the importance of consistency, it is necessary to adopt one approach among everyone who is with your kid, not five similar but not identical approaches.

These approaches are helpful through older ages, but can be used as early as two. The books have some specific guidelines for time-outs—for example, they should be shorter at younger ages and do not start until after a tantrum has ended. And they do outline some key components that are useful for very small children. For example, do not let your child use a tantrum to get what they want.

The evidence that these work is based on a number of randomized controlled trials.

To give an example, a paper published in 2003 in the *Journal of Child and Adolescent Psychiatry* reported on an evaluation of 1-2-3 Magic among 222 families.[1] All the parents involved were looking for help managing their children's behavior, although none of the children had clinical behavior problems. That is to say, they were just engaging in the standard difficult behaviors.

The intervention was fairly light—parents attended three two-hour meetings that discussed the 1-2-3 Magic approach, and were shown videos and given handouts about particular problem issues. There was a fourth two-hour meeting a month later to reinforce.

The experimental group—the one that got the intervention—had improvements on all the variables measured. The parents scored better on measures of parenting—i.e., "Are you hostile and angry toward your child?"—and the children scored better on a variety of measures of behavior. Moreover, the parents reported that their children were better behaved and more compliant, and that their own stress had gone down. The authors noted the effect sizes were not enormous—it would be hard to expect huge effects, given how limited the intervention was—but they were large enough for parents to notice them and affect their time with their children.

Smaller trials of 1-2-3 Magic with longer follow-ups have shown similar impacts, with authors arguing that the effects of these programs can be seen even two years later.[2]

The evidence isn't limited to 1-2-3 Magic. A number of studies—especially in the UK and Ireland—have seen similar impacts with the Incredible Years approach. The results there show improvements in parenting practices, reductions in child behavior problems, and lower parental stress.[3] Reviews that pull together evidence on all programs of this type show similarly consistent findings across studies. The bottom line is, they just seem to work.[4]

So, okay, these approaches work. But should you use one?

One answer to this is that it depends on the alternative. I'll talk about spanking in a bit, but the evidence suggests that it has negative consequences in both the short and long term. So if hitting is the alternative, then one of these programs is probably worth a try. And if you are tired and frustrated and feel you don't like your kid very much, then, well, that's also a reason to try.

In this way, these programs are not unlike sleep training. Many of the benefits are to the parents: lower stress, better relationship with your child, etc. (In this case, there may be some benefits at school also.) If what you are doing is working for you, great. If not, this might be worth a try.

These programs all focus on limiting disruptive behaviors—whining, fighting, tantrums, talking back—and encouraging broadly cooperative behavior like sitting at dinner and getting ready in the morning.

What about the more annoying things? Like, say, your kid insisting on singing the same song fifty times in a row? Just as an example.

You probably need to live with those. One of the main tenets of these parenting approaches is that discipline should be reserved for actual bad behavior, not for things that are merely annoying. At least one of the books I read on this suggested earplugs. It is worth noting that for an older kid, if they know you are annoyed, they'll probably do whatever annoying thing they're doing more.

It would be remiss of me to close this chapter without mentioning spanking. Although this has become a less common punishment over time, a large share of American families (estimates suggest at least half)[5] do use spanking or other forms of mild corporal punishment to address misbehavior. Some schools also still use corporal punishment.

I try, throughout this book and in my own parenting, to be truly evidence based and let the data lead me. But in this case I want to be up-front about my biases: I do not believe in spanking. There is nothing I could read in the data that would lead me to think it is a good idea, either. My impression of the data—detailed below—is that it is not, in fact, a good idea. But I want to be clear that I am starting from a place of bias.

Most studies of spanking focus on the impacts on behavior and school performance: Does spanking your child lead to more behavior problems later? Does it lead to lower school performance?

There are at least two reasons why this is a difficult question to answer with data. First, parents who spank are different from those who do not. Since many of the factors that correlate with spanking also correlate with worse outcomes for other reasons, if you look at just the raw correlation between spanking and later outcomes, you'll overstate the downside.

Second, even within the group of parents who spank, it stands to reason that children who are more difficult may be spanked more. Let's say you measure spanking behavior at age three and outcomes at age five. The data may well show (in fact, does show) that spanking at three implies more behavior problems at five. But behavior problems at three may lead to both spanking and behavior problems later. This is difficult, although perhaps not impossible, to address.

The most careful studies of this try to follow children through early childhood and look at all the possible pathways of effect. An example is a paper in *Child Development* that uses samples of almost four thousand children observed from at least age one through age five.[6] The authors looked at data on spanking at ages one, three, and five and on behavior at those ages. They tried to fully adjust for the possible pathways. For example, they correlated spanking at age one with behavior problems at age five and then asked whether that relationship goes away if you, say, control for spanking at age three.

The authors argued that spanking does have negative long-term impacts, especially on behavior problems. Spanking at age one increased behavior problems at three, and spanking at three increased behavior problems at five. These results held even with controls for earlier behavior—spanking at three relates to behavior problems at five, even controlling for behavior problems at three.

Other studies that try to carefully match families who spank to those who do not on some characteristics (income, education) similarly find spanking results in worse behavior problems.[7] Review articles on this topic similarly find small, but persistent, negative impacts on behavior.[8] There is some literature that even argues that spanking is associated with very long-term problems—alcohol abuse, suicide attempts—although it is very hard to argue this convincingly, given the other differences in family background for children who were spanked versus those who were not.[9]

There is correspondingly *no evidence* that spanking improves behavior. The same goes for other forms of physical punishment, which show evidence of negative impacts and no evidence of positive impacts.

Kids can be frustrating and, yes, they do need to be punished sometimes. But this punishment should be part of a system of discipline that aims to teach them how to be productive adults. Learning that if you misbehave you'll lose some privileges or some fun experience is something that will serve you well as an adult. Kids do not need to learn that if you misbehave, a stronger person will hit you.

The Bottom Line

- There are a variety of programs that have been shown to improve children's behavior. These focus on consistent rewards and punishments, and avoiding parental anger.
  - Examples include 1-2-3 Magic and the Incredible Years, among others.
- Spanking has not been shown to improve behavior and, indeed, has been associated with worse behavior in the short term and even through adulthood.

Education

When Finn was two he started going to preschool near where we live in Providence. It was a great place, with loving teachers and all kinds of fun stuff—a lady who spoke Spanish with puppets, an outdoor play area, "Story Time with Miss Suzanne." The school had a wonderful curriculum, one that focused on learning to share, interacting with other children, and developing a love of books. What it did not feature were classes in social studies.

Shortly before he turned three, we went on a brief sabbatical to California, where we enrolled him in a different preschool. It was also very nice, and Finn will be happy anywhere where there is a pretend kitchen, so it worked for him. But in contrast to Providence, this school seemed to be making an effort to at least pretend the two-year-olds were enrolled in a classroom for much older children. For example, they adopted an outer-space theme. The end-of-the-day message encouraged us to ask Finn, "Where do rockets go?" (Answer: "Outer space!")

With a six-month-old, trying to teach them facts about the world—or anything about letters or numbers, for example—will seem obviously fruitless. With a five-year-old, it's clearly not. At early school age, most kids are able to learn letters, some simple reading, and some math. There remains debate, which I won't get into here, about whether there is too much learning in kindergarten and whether we should be more like Finland and not teach kids to read until seven. However, if you do want to teach a five-year-old these things, you can often make some progress.

But what about a two- or three-year-old? Are there ways to set them up for academic success at this age? Is this my child's window of opportunity to learn where rockets go? If they don't, will they be behind all the children who did learn that?

These questions are really the purview of developmental psychologists, and there are some excellent books on child brain development that will do a much more comprehensive job than I can do here. *What's Going On in There?*, for example, is a great primer on how the baby and toddler brain develops. Here I'm going to focus on a limited set of questions.

First, you might have noticed that there is a lot of focus on the benefits of reading to your child. In Rhode Island, for example, the state actually gives you a new book at each well-child visit in an effort to promote reading. Tennessee sends kids a book each month (thanks to an effort spearheaded by Dolly Parton). Why do they do this, and is there any evidence that it works?

Second, beyond just reading to them, should you actively try to teach your child letters or numbers at this age? Can a two- or three-year-old actually learn to read *on their own*?

Finally, to the extent that your child does go to preschool in this age range, does it matter what kind of preschool it is? We've already been over the importance of quality in the chapter on day care, but beyond having loving teachers and a safe environment, should you care about the philosophy of the program, or even whether it has one?

READING TO YOUR CHILD

We can begin with a well-established fact. There is a large body of literature showing that children whose parents read to them as babies and preschoolers have better performance on reading tests later.[1] However, one should have significant concerns that this relationship is just a correlation, not a causal link. As we know, there are a host of factors that influence reading readiness. One of those factors is having more resources. If you're struggling to make ends meet and working two jobs, you may not have time to read to your children. Kids in this situation may also be disadvantaged in other ways.

One good way to learn something more convincing would be a randomized trial. For example, beginning with a sample of people who, perhaps, do not plan to read much to their child, you can encourage half of them to read to their child more. There are only a few small interventions of this type, most of which do not follow children long enough to evaluate impacts on test scores.[2]

One recent example is a study that used a video information program with parents to encourage "positive parenting"—specifically, reading aloud and playing—when the kids were infants to age three.[3] The authors found improvements in behavior among children whose parents watched the video, providing some suggestive evidence of the role of reading in behavior. But the data doesn't (yet) extend to school age, so we don't know the long-term effects.

In the absence of randomized evidence, researchers have tried to learn about this with other types of data. A published paper in *Child Development* in 2018 tried to use within-family variation to study this question.[4] Their basic insight was that if you have only one child, you read more to them (since you have more time). The longer you wait to have a second child, the more extra reading time the first child gets. Their idea was to compare achievement across first children with varying lengths of time before the second child arrived.

Of course, you should worry that the choice of when to have a second child is not random—this is true—but the authors have a few strategies to try to get around this, notably comparing women who intended to have a child at the same time but differed in when it happened.

The results show large positive impacts of reading on children's achievement. Children who are read to more as young children achieve greater reading success in school. One concern is that these kids just generally get more attention; this is a possibility, but the effects do not extend to math, so the authors argued that it does seem to be something about reading in particular.

There is also some neat new evidence from brain scans that help us think a bit about the cognitive effects of reading to children. In one example, researchers took nineteen children aged three to five and put them in a functional MRI (fMRI) machine.[5] In general, fMRI studies are designed to use the technology to look at which parts of the brain light up (i.e., are activated/in use) when some stimulus is provided.

In this particular study, the kids were put in the fMRI machine and then were read stories. What the researchers found was that children who were read to more at home showed more brain activation in the areas of the brain thought to be responsible for narrative processing and imagery. Basically, it looked like kids who were read to more were processing the story more effectively. How this links to later reading is unclear, and the study was small (fMRI scans are really expensive to run). Nevertheless, it provides some further evidence on the mechanisms that might drive effects.

This all suggests that reading to your child is probably a good idea. This literature goes further and actually provides some guidance on how to read to your child. In particular, researchers have found that the benefits are bigger with more interactive reading.[6] Rather than just reading a book, kids benefit from being asked open-ended questions:

"Where do you think the bird's mother is?"

"Do you think it hurts Pop when the kids hop on him?"

"How do you think the Cat in the Hat is feeling now?"

LEARNING TO READ

Reading to your child is one thing. Asking them questions is definitely something you can do. But should you go further? Should you actually try to teach your preschooler to read? Is it even possible?

Some people would say yes.

There is, for example, the Teach Your Baby to Read system,[7] which promises that you can teach your baby to read starting at around three months. You use an expensive system of flash cards and DVDs to accomplish this goal. If you doubt the success, the website suggests, just search YouTube for "baby reading," and you'll see that it is possible!

The last chapter made clear that your baby cannot learn from DVDs. It is perhaps not surprising to learn, then, that this system—which relies heavily on video—also cannot teach your child to read. Randomized evaluations using children aged nine to eighteen months show no impact of these media systems on babies' ability to read.[8] The researchers noted that this lack of success is despite parents saying that the system is very successful, suggesting that it is easy to trick yourself into thinking your child can read at a year old.

In conclusion, your baby cannot read.

On the other hand, we know that some children aged four to five *can* read, and studies that focus on this age group show, for example, that it is possible to actively teach four-year-olds letter sounds and the idea of blending them into words.[9] If you are inclined to teach your four-year-old to read, you can probably make some progress. There is a separate question of whether you want to, but that is more a parenting choice than a question for the data.

A two- or three-year-old, though . . . They are not a baby, but they are not a five-year-old. Your just-three-year-old can talk and, sometimes, understand what you are asking him to do. It seems plausible, but not certain, that he could learn to read.

The truth is that there is not much literature on extremely early reading. There are some examples—case reports—of children who learn to read fluently at very young ages—two and a half, early three.[10] The children in these reports have prodigy-level reading. They are not just reading "Mat sat" at three—they are reading at a third-grade level. And in most of these cases, it is clear the child more or less just picked up reading on their own. Their parents were not sitting and teaching them to sound out *C-A-R*.

Children who learn to read like this—and this is also true of kids who learn to read early within the normal range—are more likely to learn with sight words than phonics. They tend to have a larger share of their reading involve recognition rather than sounding out. Interestingly, early readers are not necessarily good spellers.

It should be said that some cases of this prodigious early reading are associated with autism. Hyperlexia (as it is called) is a trait of some high-functioning autistic children; children can read but do not understand.[11]

What there simply isn't evidence on is whether you can teach a two- or three-year-old the letter sounds and some early phonics. If you try to engage in the same approach you'd take with a four-year-old, will it work? The data doesn't have an answer. Anecdotally (I know, I know—no anecdotes), you do see kids this age who know their letter sounds, but rarely ones who read full books on their own. If you want your child to know that *S* says *"Sssss,"* you can probably do that. They're likely not going to be reading Harry Potter, though.

TYPES OF PRESCHOOL

At some point, around the age of two or three, you may start thinking of childcare as closer to "school." If your child is home with a parent or nanny, this is an age at which people often explore part-time "preschool" options, designed (in general) to increase socialization, and possibly to start teaching school-type skills. If your child is in day care, their older classrooms will often be a more structured form of school.

Let's ask the first question: Is it a good idea to put your child in preschool?

We can look for some evidence on this by thinking back to the chapter on day care. The evidence I discussed there showed that more time in day care after eighteen months or so was associated with better language and literacy development at slightly later ages. This is about the best evidence we have that preschool might be a good idea.

There is also evidence from small and much older randomized trials suggesting that programs like Head Start improve school readiness. But these tend to focus on enrollment at older ages—say, four—and on especially disadvantaged populations.

Putting this together, it again probably depends on the other options for your child during the day, but I'd say the weight of the evidence is that some preschool environment around age two or three will, on average, improve the ease with which they transition to school.

Having decided you want to try some preschool, the question is then, which one? Again, we can hark back to the day care chapter. Day care and preschool at this age are distinguishable largely by the length of time: people tend to think of "preschool" as a half-day activity and "day care" as an all-day activity. Still, if you look at many day-care programs at this age, they tend to have a more preschool-like morning session and then a nap-and-play afternoon session.

This means that many of the "quality" measures we discussed in the day care section apply here, too—is the area safe, do the adults seem engaged, etc.

When we start to talk about preschools, people do begin to ask questions like, Is it important that the teachers be trained in early childhood development? Or, going further, does it matter *where* they trained? We simply do not have reasonable evidence on this. Preschool teachers vary in quality—you can see this in any preschool you go to—but the data simply is not sufficient to tell us to look for something like quality of teacher training.

A related question is whether you should favor one preschool "philosophy" over others. The three philosophies you will most commonly encounter in your preschool exploration are Montessori, Reggio Emilia, and Waldorf.

Montessori education focuses on a particular classroom structure and a set of materials. There is an emphasis—even in young children—on the development of fine motor skills. These schools generally refer to children's play as "works." Young children are typically exposed to letters and numbers and writing them in sand, counting blocks, and so on.

Reggio Emilia–inspired schools put more emphasis on play, with typically little formal letter or number exposure at preschool ages. (One Reggio Emilia–style preschool I visited told me they explicitly do not spend any time on letters for the three- and four-year-old class, and wouldn't even display letter cards around the room. This seemed a little extreme.)

The Waldorf schools have a heavy outdoor component and, similar to Reggio Emilia, are largely play-based. The Waldorf principles focus on learning through play and art, and tend to also have some domestic-activity component (cooking, baking, gardening).

All three methods have a structured day, so kids know what to expect when. They all acknowledge that young kids benefit from being able to explore in a safe environment and to self-direct, to some extent, in what they do.

I cannot do justice here to the full philosophy in each. Many books have been written on these methods, and implementation varies significantly across individual schools. Montessori is most consistent—if you visit a bunch of Montessori classrooms, as I did on a whirlwind cross-country job search when Penelope was three, you'll find some strong similarities in the materials they use and the structure of the day. However, there are still wide differences, probably having mostly to do with the inclinations and skills of the staff. You'll find many schools describing themselves as "Reggio Emilia–inspired," which could mean strongly inspired or loosely inspired or just a teeny bit inspired.

And, of course, not all preschools will have one of these particular philosophies. A lot of preschools may pull lessons from one or the other of these groups, but do not strictly adhere to all their approaches. And many preschools also have a religious connection or affiliation, which will affect their curriculum.

Is one of these better than the others? There are clearly quality differences across preschools, but this isn't the same as saying that one philosophy dominates.

Unfortunately, there is again really not much evidence on this— especially not of the type that would be relevant to people who are already thinking carefully about the optimal preschool philosophy. To the extent that there is any evidence at all, it's mostly on Montessori education, since this is a popular and established approach.

There are some studies showing the children in Montessori preschools perform better on reading and math tests compared to a control group in non-Montessori options.[12] But many of the papers on this are very old, and it's not clear that early learning of reading and math skills are the main goals of preschool education.

Indeed, the non-Montessori approaches often emphasize the importance of play and argue that early literacy is not an important outcome. Proponents of this argument will often point to Finland, where (famously) most children attend a state-run kindergarten that does not attempt to teach reading fluency. Kids learn to read starting in first grade (although, realistically, some of them do read before that). These proponents will also commonly note that Finland performs very well on international standardized tests—much better than the US—and argue that this means we may put too much emphasis on the value of early literacy.

The fact that Finland performs better than the US is not a helpful observation, in my view, since many places perform better than the US on these tests. This includes many countries in Asia with much more rigorous early-life instruction.

And the actual evidence on the relative value of this approach is thin. There are a couple of non-randomized studies from outside the US showing that children who learn to read later do catch up in terms of reading within a few years and that teaching the alphabet early doesn't necessarily impact reading.[13] But on the other hand, we know that programs like

Head Start, which focus on early literacy, do improve school performance early on.

All this is to say that, again, we simply do not have a lot of concrete data to guide you. Further complicating both research and decision-making, it is possible—even likely—that the best type of preschool will vary by individual child. If your kid struggles to sit still, they may find an environment focused on fine motor skills to be taxing; on the other hand, it may be good for them. So it may really be useless to try to learn what is best for your kid from a study—even a good one—that estimates the effect of a type of preschool for the average child.

The Bottom Line

- There is some support for the value of reading to your children starting in infancy.
- Your baby cannot learn to read. Whether your two- or three-year-old can is unclear, but it would be very unusual for them to be a fluent reader.
- Evidence on the value of different preschool philosophies is limited.

PART FOUR

The Home Front

This is a book about babies and small children. But it cannot escape our notice that when a baby arrives it also magically creates parents. This is not always easy. Indeed, there are books written about the "transition to parenthood," and they are not all filled with the adorable pictures you see on your friends' Facebook feeds.

Becoming a parent is challenging. I think in some ways it is more challenging for this generation than the last. On one hand, we have a lot of stuff they didn't (disposable diapers, Amazon Prime). On the other hand, as people have children later, when their careers and lifestyles are already more established, the challenge of adaptation is harder.

There is adaptation for parents individually, and adaptation together. *How does this baby fit into the plans I have for myself, for my career, for my leisure time? And how does it fit into our marriage?*

For the most part, data and evidence will probably not help with these transitions, as they are different for everyone. The goal of this part of the book is not so much to tell you what to do (indeed, I will have no advice at all), but rather to acknowledge that we should be talking about what works for the family, not just what works for the baby.

The bottom line—perhaps the most important in this book—is that parents are people, too. Having a kid doesn't make you stop being a person with needs and desires and ambitions. It almost certainly changes those, but it doesn't eliminate them. Being a good parent isn't about completely subsuming your entire personhood into your children. In fact, if you let your kids rule, it can have the opposite effect.

We talked some about these issues when we covered the choice about parental work outside of the home in part 2 of the book. Here I'll pick that back up and talk about at least some of the challenges with the transition to parenthood, and with thinking about growing your family.

Internal Politics

When you change something substantial about your relationship with your partner, there is bound to be some conflict. For example, the first time you live together—at least for most couples—has its moments of tension.

When I first moved in with Jesse, I recall a deep and lasting conflict over kitchen sponge etiquette. He believes you should wring out the sponge and place it next to the sink when done using it. I take a more laissez-faire approach to the sponge, preferring to let it lie where it falls in the sink. It drove him crazy when he'd come to the sink hours after I'd been there to find a still wet and now smelly sponge soaking in its own juices.

Ultimately, we fixed this by some combination of my attempts to improve (although before I sat down to write this chapter, I noticed I had left the sponge in the sink, soaking wet, the night before, so obviously I have not improved much in fifteen years) and his attempts to let it go (even though he is objectively correct about the right thing to do in this case). The most important change was probably the decision to have him do the dishes. I am proud to say it has been years since we have had any sponge-related conflict.

Introducing a child into your life will, similarly, lead to some increase in tension for most people. Less charitably, people will tell you that children will "ruin your marriage."

It is easy to see why this might be. You and your partner both want the best thing for your child—indeed, you want this more than anything you've ever wanted. However, most of the time you have no idea what this "best thing" is. And you'll sometimes disagree, either due to deep underlying differences or simply because you both have no idea and your best guesses differ.

Obviously, you've disagreed about things before (sponges, for example). But on the whole, these disagreements were not as important, and there were not as many of them. The worst thing that happens with a wet sponge is you have to replace it. But if you mess up your kid, that's forever! The stakes seem infinitely high.

And at the same time, you're exhausted and you have less money and less time. Jesse and I dated, and lived together, for almost a decade before Penelope arrived. We were used to having control of our own time, to spending the weekends in some combination of working (him), writing (me), sewing (me), going to brunch, seeing friends. Now, all of a sudden, the weekend was a haze of feeding, dealing with poop, attempting to shower, holding a screaming baby at brunch with friends, not sleeping, waiting anxiously for the nanny to arrive Monday morning. It was great, and I wouldn't trade it for anything—even at the time—but there is no question that nerves fray more quickly and conflicts can worsen fast in this situation.

So it does seem like—based on logic—kids could stress your marriage. And if you look on the internet, you'll definitely find some people who think it does. They write articles with titles like "You Will Hate Your Husband After Your Kid Is Born (Don't Let Anyone Tell You Otherwise)."[1] But these are just examples—anecdotes. Some people clearly do hate their partner after their kids arrive. Of course, some people also hate their partner *before* kids. Are things systematically worse after kids arrive? And is there anything you can do about it?[2]

The answer to the first question is yes, things are, on average, systematically worse in marriages after kids. It is probably an exaggeration to say you'll "hate your spouse," but people (women in particular) do seem less happy after kids.

We can see this in a variety of studies that look at the relationship between parenthood and marital satisfaction. These go back as early as 1970, with a paper showing that between the pre-childbearing period and the period of having school-aged children, the share of mothers reporting low marital satisfaction rises gradually from 12 percent to 30 percent, with an abrupt jump in the first year of the child's life. The marriage does not recover until parents become grandparents.[3]

Meta-analyses of more recent data show similar things—parents are less happy with their marriages than nonparents. The changes seem to be most abrupt in the first year, and then there is some recovery, although not complete.[4] As one study helpfully notes, "In sum, parenthood hastens marital decline. . . ."[5]

It is worth noting that these studies do tend to find that people who are happier before they have kids recover better, and that planned pregnancies are less impactful than unplanned ones. And the effects are not enormously large. Many people are still, on net, happy with their spouse. Just, you know, slightly less.

Why is this? It is, of course, hard to know, and probably varies across couples. One issue may simply be the lack of time to focus on the relationship. Before you have children, your relationship is just about the two of you—you have the luxury of sleeping late together, going out, just spending hours talking about what is going on, big and small. Once you have kids, it is almost impossible to replicate this, and if you are not careful, you can find that you virtually never talk about anything other than the children. The relationship falls by the wayside, and not usually for the better. You're connected through your children, but it can feel like you've lost the connection to your partner.

Being aware of this may be helpful, and in this chapter I talk about some proposed solutions to the marital-happiness problems. But before doing that, it's useful to look at two specific things that researchers have speculated play a role in the marital-happiness decline. The first is unequal chore allocation: women tend to do the bulk of household work, even if they also work outside the home. The second is a decline in sex: parents have less sex, and sex makes people happy.

Is there evidence for either of these? Broadly, yes.

Beginning with the basic facts: If we look at time-use data—that is, people's reports of how much time they spend on various activities—we see that, on average, women spend more time than men on housework and child-rearing-related activities. Even if we compare women who work full time with men who work full time, the women spend about an hour and a half more during the day caring for kids, doing housework, and shopping.[6]

The amount of time women spend on these activities has declined a lot over time (thanks, washing machines/dishwashers/microwaves!), but it is still unequal.[7] And it's notable that women do more housework even if they also make more money. When women bring in more than 90 percent of the household income, they still do almost as much housework as the men in these households. In contrast, when men bring in more than 90 percent of household income, they do much less housework.[8]

An interesting question (at least for an economist) is whether this lack of equality is unavoidable. One theory is that many household tasks cannot be divided up, so one person has to do more of them, and it ends up being the female partner due to some small underlying skill differences. For example, maybe women are inherently better at cooking as adults because they are more likely to have been taught to cook as children.

This would be a version of an economic theory of comparative advantage. This explanation would rely, among other things, on the assumption that it is not possible or efficient to divide the tasks equally.

That doesn't seem to be the case. One piece of data comes from comparisons across countries and over time; in Sweden, for example, the household work is split more evenly.[9] And over time, even in the US, it has gotten more equal, as we've moved away (to some extent) from traditional gender roles.

Also within the US, we have some (limited) evidence from same-sex couples, which shows that they share household work more equally than different-sex couples.[10] These samples tend to be small, so any results should be taken with a grain of salt, but they are suggestive.

Of course, the basic fact of lack of equality doesn't translate to dissatisfaction, but there is yet more data—again, from surveys—suggesting that this lack of equality is a source of unhappiness and tension for women.[11] Indeed, we certainly see a fair amount of anecdotal evidence that women resent the idea of a "second shift," and that it crowds out leisure time, which men end up with more of. Indeed, there are whole books written on this dynamic and the problems it creates.[12]

So chores are one problem. What about lack of sex?

Again, it is well documented that parents have less sex.[13] This is especially true in the first months or year after childbirth, but generally, data shows that couples have less sex after they have children than before. It is easy to see why this might be—less time, more exhaustion, other people (i.e., the children) in your bed.

As with household-work time, the fact that this is true isn't necessarily a problem. If both partners want to have sex less frequently, then this change may be fine. This doesn't seem to be the case for many couples, but we do not have a lot of systematic data beyond anecdote. Certainly, anecdotes would suggest that people on both sides of the relationship, although more men than women, would like to have more sex, and find the reduction in sex frequency to be difficult for the relationship.

Although it may be surprising, there is speculation (at least on the internet) that these sources of unhappiness are linked. If men do more chores, do you have more sex?

You may be surprised to learn that there is robust, if not especially good, academic literature on this relationship. In fact, the effects go both ways. Some studies suggest that if men do more chores, the couple has less sex. Some suggest the opposite—that the couple has more sex.[14] Generally, these findings come from surveys in which people are asked about what share of chores they do and about the frequency with which they have sex.

Theories for why these links would occur abound. On the "more chores, less sex" side, people argue that seeing a man wash the dishes is emasculating and a turnoff for women. On the "more chores, more sex" side, people argue that seeing a man wash the dishes is a turn-on—plus, if men do more work, it frees up more time for women, meaning more time for sex!

In fact, I think a much better theory is that these are not causally linked in either direction, and research that finds a link is confused by missing variables. People in happier marriages probably have more sex, but also may share chores more equally. This would lead to a positive sex–chore relationship, but it's really just marital happiness overall. On the other hand, when both people work, they may have less sex because they have less time, but they also may share chores more equally. This would lead to a negative sex–chore relationship, but it's really just about working.

Since these biases go in both directions, it's virtually impossible to learn anything.

It may be good to get your spouse to do the dishes, but the value of that is that the dishes get done, not that you're going to be inspired to start ripping their clothes off in a haze of soap suds and flying plates.

SOLUTIONS

It's all well and good to say the data says kids ruin your marriage. But are there solutions other than waiting until you have grandchildren to be happy again?

Although it is not a solution, it is worth noting that couples who are happier in their marriage before kids and who planned their pregnancies tend to have smaller declines and faster rebounds in their happiness.

The second thing to say is that, as is a common refrain in this book, sleep is a key issue.[15] Drops in marital satisfaction are higher in couples with kids who sleep less. Lack of parental sleep contributes to depression (in both parents) and correspondingly to less-happy marriages. You need sleep to function, and sleep deprivation affects your mood. If you are cranky, you're cranky with your partner. If they are also tired, they are also cranky. Cranky, cranky, sad, angry.

Can you fix this? It's hard early on, but see the earlier chapter on sleep training as one solution. Even if this particular approach isn't for you, thinking carefully about ways you might improve the adult sleep in the house is worth some time.

Beyond the role of sleep—and pushing out of infancy—we do not have a lot of evidence on what works to improve marriages. Indeed, if I had better evidence on that, I could write another book on it.

Some small-scale randomized interventions do show some effectiveness. One is the "marriage checkup."[16] The idea behind this is to have an annual meeting—possibly facilitated by some professional—to actually discuss your marriage. What do you feel is working? What isn't working? Are there particular areas of concern or unhappiness? These checkups seem to result in improvements in intimacy (i.e., sex) and marital satisfaction. This makes sense in the abstract; it's helpful to talk things through methodically with a neutral third party.

Beyond this particular intervention, there is other evidence in favor of therapy more generally—group couples therapy, counseling programs beginning before birth and continuing after—to improve relationships.[17] Speaking in broad generalizations, these focus on communication and positive solutions to conflict.

Part of the reason these work may simply be that they force both people in the household to reflect on what the other person is doing for the family. You can see the things you are doing clearly, and you probably have some sense of what your partner does, but you do not always see it so obviously.

One of Jesse's jobs in our house is taking out the trash—both collecting and taking it from the house and, especially, taking it to the curb on

Mondays. I had always thought of this as a relatively simple task that didn't deserve much credit. Then one day he was gone on a Monday, and he sent me this email.

From: Jesse

To: Emily

Subject: Trash Instructions

Taking trash out

- Tie up bin liner in trash
- Roll trash out to street, make sure to leave room for recycling
- Roll recycling out to street
- Make sure there is room between the two bins so they can lift them separately

Taking trash back in

- Roll bins back to their area
- Recycling goes in first, closest to garage
- Then trash goes
- Put some diatomaceous earth in trash and recycling
- Put some baking soda if there is an odor
- Put a new bin liner (in mud room closet) in trash (not in recycling)

Then congratulations you are done!

Apparently, due to some maggot and fly issues (I have a problem with bugs, but also tend to do things that attract them, like failing to fully close the garbage bags), he had adopted a many-step system involving something called "diatomaceous earth" to keep things dry and bug-free.

I was sorry to have to do this at all, but it made me a lot more grateful for the 99 percent of Mondays that he does it.

The Bottom Line

- Marital satisfaction does decline, on average, after children.
- These declines are smaller and briefer if you're happier before children, and if the kids are planned.
- Unequal division of labor and less sex probably do play some role, although it is hard to get a sense of how important these are.
- There is some small-scale evidence suggesting marital counseling and "marriage checkup" programs can improve happiness.

20

Expansions

S ome people have told me they are ready for another baby on leaving the delivery room. Others take years before reluctantly wanting to try again. Some never want another kid. Some people plan out the child timing precisely—down to the month. Others adopt more of a wait-and-see approach.

This chapter is about the choice of whether to have more than one child, and, if you decide to have another child, the choice of timing. Is there an "optimal" number of children? Or an ideal spacing between them?

Spoiler alert: There isn't much of a science-based answer to these questions. Any small impacts are likely to be dramatically outweighed by the most important consideration, which is what works for your family.

For example, if you have your first child at thirty-eight and you want three kids, you'll likely have to have them pretty quickly. If you're a doctor and you are planning your kids around residency, this will tell you your timing. And, of course, things change. You do not always get pregnant when you want to. Due to a lack of maternity leave, my mom attempted to time my brother to arrive over Christmas break, but she got January 11 instead.

Sometimes life intervenes. I thought we'd have our kids closer in age—more like three years apart, rather than four. But then I had a big, and unexpected, professional setback right around when we'd need to start working on number two. I was barely in emotional shape to parent one kid, never mind have another. So we waited.

The choice of how many children to have is even more personal. Does your family feel done with just one? Do you want another? And, of course, sometimes it's hard to have a second child, and sometimes it's an accident.

All this is to say that the data has very little to add to your family preferences. But we can visit the data there is, first on the question of number of children, and then—conditional on the number—the question of birth spacing.

NUMBER OF CHILDREN

Economists are very interested in number of children and, beginning with Gary Becker's influential work, in the "quantity-quality" trade-off. The idea here is that parents face a tension between number and quality of kids. If you have more kids, then you cannot invest as much in each of them, so they'll be "lower quality."

By "quality," we tend to mean things like school attainment—the "investments" you make as a parent are in your child's education, IQ, etc. Let no one tell you economists are not clinical about their discussions of parenting.

Much of the economic writing about this focuses on understanding what is called the "demographic transition"—the movement of countries as they develop from very high fertility rates (think: six to eight kids) to lower (two or three). The idea is that as your country gets richer, you might want to focus on quality of children rather than quantity, and this would drive some of these fertility declines.

The basic theory that there is a quantity-quality trade-off would imply that if you have more kids, they will do worse in terms of human capital—less education, maybe lower IQ. But this is just a theory—what does the data say?

As with most things in the book, this is difficult to test, since the kinds of parents who have many children differ from those who have few. But some researchers have done this, generally using a method with "surprise" births. They look at the arrival of twins as something that increases the size of the family while not affecting the number of children you actually wanted.[1]

The results from the best of these papers generally show that the number of children plays a relatively little role in determining schooling or IQ.[2] They do find that birth order matters. Later-born children tend to do (slightly) worse on IQ tests and get less schooling than their earlier-born siblings. This may be due to parents having less time and resources to devote to them. But it's not the number of children that drives the association. A firstborn child with two siblings seems to do the same as a firstborn child with one.[3]

A second question people (typically not economists) often ask is whether there is some downside to having an only child—will they be socially awkward?

Again, this is hard to study, given the differences across families. To the extent that we have evidence, this concern seems unfounded. One review article, which summarizes 140 studies on this broad question, found some evidence of more "academic motivation" among only children, but no differences in personality traits like extroversion.[4] Even this fact about academic motivation may be more about birth order—firstborn children score higher on this regardless of whether they have siblings—than about being an only child.

Based on such paltry data, it is hard to say with confidence that it doesn't matter how many children you have. And your kids' relationships with their siblings (if you choose to have them) will define many things about them—for good and for ill. But there isn't anything in the data that would tell you one choice is necessarily better than another.

BIRTH SPACING

So let's say you decide you want to have another kid. Does the data tell you when you should do it?

Again, no, not really. To the extent research has been done on "optimal birth spacing," it tends to focus on two things: the relationship between birth spacing and infant health, and the relationship between birth spacing and long-term outcomes like school performance and IQ.

Most of the discussion focuses on distinguishing more typical birth intervals (say, two to four years apart) from very short ones (less than eighteen months) or very long (more than five years). However, regardless of the outcome you are studying, this is a challenging data problem. The issue is that both very short and very long intervals are unusual.

Some people do plan to have two children very close together in age, but relative to other birth intervals, babies born within a year of each other are less likely to be planned. Unplanned births may have different outcomes than planned ones, even putting aside spacing. On the flip side, very long spacing between children is also somewhat unusual. It is more likely—not certain, but more likely—that families with very long birth spacing struggled with fertility challenges. This could matter as well, especially when we look at infant health.

For these reasons, we want to take most of the evidence with a grain—or, really, a big handful—of salt.

Infant Health

Studies of infant health and birth spacing tend to focus on outcomes that can be measured at birth: for example, is the child premature, low birth weight, or small for gestational age? Correlational studies have shown links between both short birth intervals and long birth intervals and all these outcomes. For example, in a 2017 study of almost 200,000 births in Canada, researchers found that there was an 83 percent increase in the risk of preterm birth for women who got pregnant within six months of their last birth.[5]

These large effects also show up in other studies—one in California and another in the Netherlands—that focused on recurrence of preterm birth (i.e., the analysis was limited to women who had already had a preterm birth).[6]

This very large effect is not, however, replicated everywhere, and there is a question of whether it might be driven by differences across moms. This concern is at least somewhat validated by a study in Sweden that was able to compare women to other women—siblings or cousins—in their family. This addresses the concern that some family-level differences are driving the results.

In comparing siblings, they were effectively asking whether two children born to the same mother have different outcomes depending on the birth interval. To the extent that we worry that some mothers differ from others, this addressed that concern.[7]

These Swedish researchers replicated the finding that very short birth intervals increase prematurity when they compared across families, but they found much smaller effects (more like 20 percent than 80 percent) when they compared siblings. The effects when comparing cousins were somewhere in the middle. They found no association between these short intervals and low birth weight or other outcomes once they compared siblings.

Although there is a lively debate about which set of numbers to believe, I think there is a good argument in favor of the sibling comparisons, which would suggest that although there is some elevated risk of prematurity with very short spacing, it is not very large.

This Swedish study does find that very long intervals—here defined as more than five years between birth and the next pregnancy—are associated with worse outcomes. And we see some similar evidence in the

Canadian work. However, very long intervals between births are unusual, and more likely to be associated with older mothers or fertility problems. It is not clear how much we want to learn from this about *choosing* longer intervals.

Long-Run Outcomes

Infant health is important but short term. Are there any long-run consequences for children related to birth spacing? Are test scores lower for children whose siblings are close in age?

This analysis is challenging since people choose their birth spacing, to some degree. But at least one study tried to compare women who intended to have babies at the same time but ended up having them at different times (for example, due to miscarriage).[8]

When researchers performed this analysis, they found that for the older child, test scores were higher if there was more space between that child and their younger sibling. This may reflect, for example, more parental time invested in reading or other skill development at young ages. These effects, though, were pretty small.

For these younger children, at times concerns have been raised about links between short birth spacing and autism.[9] Although multiple studies of this do show some links, they are not able to adjust as well for differences across families, so this evidence remains suggestive.

Overall, what do we take from all this? I would argue that any links there are are not consistent or large enough to outweigh the preferences that you are likely to have.

To the extent that you have no preferences at all about this, I think the bulk of the evidence suggests there are some small risks—both short and possibly long term—to very short birth intervals. So waiting until the first child is at least a year old to get pregnant again may be a good idea. It also just may be easier on you as a parent, given the intensity of the infant stage.

The Bottom Line

- The data doesn't provide much guidance about the ideal number of children or birth interval between them.
- There may be some risks to very short intervals, including preterm birth and (possibly) higher rates of autism.

21

Growing Up and Letting Go

When Penelope was almost three and we were thinking about having a second kid, Jesse and I were also in the job market, looking for two faculty jobs together. We went to Michigan, where we were invited to the house of two slightly older economists whose children were fifteen and eighteen. The conversation about economics exhausted, we turned to talking about our kids.

"The thing is," one of them told us, "when our kids were four and one, we used to look at each other and say, 'I can't wait until they are in high school and everything will be easy.' Then finally, last year, they were both in high school, and what we learned is that there is no problem that cannot be solved with a four-hour discussion every night about the minute details of high-school social life."

When you're in the thick of it with very early parenting—with the exhaustion and uncertainty of it all—there is the promise in the distance of a time when your child will use the bathroom on their own, put on their own jacket, and eat with a fork. And it is definitely true that the first time my son came out of the bathroom and said he had peed on his own, I did a little jig.

But there is a flip side. Little kids mean mostly little problems. As your kid gets bigger, the number of things you worry about goes down, but they get more important. Is my kid achieving academically? Are they fitting in socially? Most important, are they happy?

Part of what makes this hard, especially for someone like me, is that the problems get more varied as kids get older, and much less amenable to data analysis. Sure, you can look at some data about whether the "new math" is better than the "old math," but how to get a child to engage socially, and whether that even matters, is largely beyond the realm of easy empirical analysis. We have to grope forward, ideally listening to our kids to see what works for them—if it takes a four-hour conversation, we'll clear our schedules.

We keep at it, in part because the rewards are correspondingly so much bigger. Seeing your kid do well at something they love, seeing them excited about learning something new, watching them work through a challenge— there is nothing better. And you do not need data to tell you that. So just remember that while there will always be parenting challenges, there are many joys on the horizon, too.

As hard as it is to believe when you're staring down preschool, your parenting adventure is still just beginning. But you certainly know more than you did back in the delivery room. Progress!

You know that early parenting is full of advice. This book, it's full of advice (or at least decision processes). As I finished writing, I therefore thought about the question, *What is the best parenting advice I've ever gotten?*

Here it is.

When Penelope was two, we planned a vacation in France with some friends. We had been to the location before and I knew there were lots of bees.

At our two-year-old well-child visit, I therefore had a set of questions for Dr. Li.

"Here's what I'm worried about. We are going on this vacation, and there are bees. It's kind of isolated. What if Penelope is stung? She's never been stung before. What if she's allergic? How will I get her to a doctor in time? Should I bring something to be prepared for this? Should we test her in advance? Do I need an EpiPen?"

Dr. Li paused. She looked at me. And then she said, very calmly:

"Hmm. I'd probably just try not to think about that."

And that's it. "Just try not to think about that." She was right, obviously. I had built up this elaborate and incredibly unlikely scenario in my head. Yes, this could all happen. But so could a million other things. Parenting cannot be about thinking about every possible eventuality, every possible misstep. Sometimes, you just need to let it go.

So, yes, it makes sense to take parenting seriously, and to want to make the best choices for your kid and the best choices for you. But there will be many times that you need to just trust that if you're doing your best, that's all you can do. Being present and happy with your kids is more important than, say, worrying about bees.

At the end, let's raise a glass to using data where it's useful, to making the right decisions for our families, to doing our best, and—sometimes—to just trying not to think about it.

ACKNOWLEDGMENTS

Thank you, first, to my wonderful agent, Suzanne Gluck, and my amazing editor, Ginny Smith. Without you two this definitely would not have gotten off the ground or finished. I am grateful to Ann Godoff and the whole team at Penguin for being willing to go around with me again on this book, and for supporting my first one so wonderfully.

Adam Davis was an incredible and patient medical editor. The book would not have come together without his advice and guidance.

Charles Wood, Dawn Li, Lauren Ward, and Ashley Larkin also provided invaluable medical commentary.

Emilia Ruzicka and Sven Ostertag contributed excellent graphical design. Xana Zhang, Ruby Steele, Lauren To, and Geoffrey Kocks provided invaluable research assistance, from literature reviews and fact checking to proofreading and paper collation.

In conception, this book benefited hugely from idea generation from many people. From the Brooklyn focus group: Meghan Weidl, Meriwether Schas, Emily Byne, Rhiannon Gulick, Hannah Gladstein, Marisa Robertson-Textor, Jax Zummo, Salma Abdelnour, Melissa Wells, Laura Ball, Lena Berger, Emily Hoch, Brooke Lewis, Alexandra Sowa, Barin Porzar, Rachel Friedman, Rebecca Youngerman, and especially Lesley Duval. And from everyone on Twitter, and the Academic Moms on Facebook.

Thank you to everyone who read and commented on drafts: Emma Berndt, Eric Budish, Heidi Williams, Michelle McClosky, Kelly Joseph,

Josh Gottleib, Carolin Pfluger, Dan Benjamin, Samantha Cherney, Emily Shapiro, and Laura Wheery.

Thanks to the girls, who read a lot of this and shared their experiences and let me use them: Jane Risen, Jenna Robins, Tricia Patrick, Divya Mathur, Elena Zinchenko, Hilary Friedman, Heather Caruso, Katie Kinzler, and Alix Morse. And most important, they were there to celebrate the good stuff and talk me through the less good stuff. I love you guys.

Many colleagues and friends supported the idea and reality of this book at various stages. Including but by no means limited to Judy Chevalier, Anna Aizer, David Weil, Matt Notowidigdo, Dave Nussbaum, Nancy Rose, Amy Finkelstein, Andrei Shleifer, Nancy Zimmerman, and the More Dudes.

A very special thanks to Matt Gentzkow, who took seriously my desire to write another book, talked me through whether it was a good idea, and provided invaluable editing. Not surprisingly, Jesse's favorite sentence in this book was written by Matt.

We have been lucky to have wonderful pediatricians in both Chicago and Rhode Island—Dawn Li and Lauren Ward—without whom parenting would be much harder. And we are also lucky to have had wonderful childcare—most of all Mardele Castel, Rebecca Shirley, and Sarah Hudson—but also the teachers at Moses Brown and the Little School at Lincoln.

My incredibly supportive family. Thank you to the Shapiros: Joyce, Arvin, and Emily. To the Fairs and Osters: Steve, Rebecca, John, and Andrea. And to my parents, Ray and Sharon. Mom, I know this makes you nervous, but thanks for supporting it anyway.

It goes without saying that without Penelope and Finn there would be no book. Thanks to Penelope for reading it, and to both of you for helping me learn to be a mom.

Jesse. Parenting is hard. I am glad I get to do it with you. Thank you for supporting me in my crazy ideas. You're a great husband, and a great father. Also, you're really good at managing the trash. I love you.

APPENDIX:

FURTHER READING

These books, which cover many of the topics discussed in this book, may be helpful further reading.

GENERAL REFERENCE

American Academy of Pediatrics. *Caring for Your Baby and Young Child: Birth to Age Five*. New York: Bantam, 2004.

Druckerman, P. *Bringing Up Bébé: One American Mother Discovers the Wisdom of French Parenting*. New York: Penguin, 2014.

Eliot, L. *What's Going On in There?: How the Brain and Mind Develop in the First Five Years of Life*. New York: Bantam, 2000.

Nathanson, L. *The Portable Pediatrician for Parents: A Month-by-Month Guide to Your Child's Physical and Behavioral Development from Birth to Age Five*. New York: Harper-Collins, 1994.

DISCIPLINE

Phelan, T. W. *1-2-3 Magic: Effective Discipline for Children 2–12*. Naperville, IL: Parent-Magic, Inc., 2010.

Webster-Stratton, C. *The Incredible Years: A Trouble-Shooting Guide for Parents of Children Aged 2–8*. Toronto: Umbrella Press, 1992.

SLEEP

Ferber, R. *Solve Your Child's Sleep Problems*. Rev. ed. New York: Simon & Schuster, 2006.

Karp, H. *The Happiest Baby on the Block: The New Way to Calm Crying and Help Your Newborn Baby Sleep Longer.* Rev. ed. New York: Bantam, 2015.

Weissbluth, M. *Healthy Sleep Habits, Happy Child: A Step-by-Step Program for a Good Night's Sleep.* 4th ed. New York: Ballantine Books, 2015.

POTTY TRAINING

Glowacki, J. *Oh Crap! Potty Training: Everything Modern Parents Need to Know to Do It Once and Do It Right.* New York: Touchstone, 2015.

NOTES

CHAPTER 1: THE FIRST THREE DAYS

1. Preer G, Pisegna JM, Cook JT, Henri AM, Philipp BL. Delaying the bath and in-hospital breastfeeding rates. *Breastfeed Med* 2013;8(6):485–90.
2. Nako Y, Harigaya A, Tomomasa T, et al. Effects of bathing immediately after birth on early neonatal adaptation and morbidity: A prospective randomized comparative study. *Pediatr Int* 2000;42(5): 517–22.
3. Loring C, Gregory K, Gargan B, et al. Tub bathing improves thermoregulation of the late preterm infant. *J Obstet Gynecol Neonatal Nurs* 2012;41(2):171–79.
4. Weiss HA, Larke N, Halperin D, Schenker I. Complications of circumcision in male neonates, infants and children: A systematic review. *BMC Urol* 2010;10:2.
5. Weiss HA et al. Complications of circumcision in male neonates, infants and children.
6. Van Howe RS. Incidence of meatal stenosis following neonatal circumcision in a primary care setting. *Clin Pediatr (Phila)* 2006;45(1):49–54.
7. Bazmamoun H, Ghorbanpour M, Mousavi-Bahar SH. Lubrication of circumcision site for prevention of meatal stenosis in children younger than 2 years old. *Urol J* 2008;5(4):233–36.
8. Bossio JA, Pukall CF, Steele S. A review of the current state of the male circumcision literature. *J Sex Med* 2014;11(12):2847–64.
9. Singh-Grewal D, Macdessi J, Craig J. Circumcision for the prevention of urinary tract infection in boys: A systematic review of randomised trials and observational studies. *Arch Dis Child* 2005;90(8): 853–58.
10. Sorokan ST, Finlay JC, Jefferies AL. Newborn male circumcision. *Paediatr Child Health* 2015;20(6): 311–20.
11. Bossio JA et al. A review of the current state of the male circumcision literature.
12. Daling JR, Madeleine MM, Johnson LG, et al. Penile cancer: Importance of circumcision, human papillomavirus and smoking in in situ and invasive disease. *Int J Cancer* 2005;116(4):606–16.
13. Taddio A, Katz J, Ilersich AL, Koren G. Effect of neonatal circumcision on pain response during subsequent routine vaccination. *Lancet* 1997;349(9052):599–603.
14. Brady-Fryer B, Wiebe N, Lander JA. Pain relief for neonatal circumcision. *Cochrane Database Syst Rev* 2004;(4):CD004217.
15. Wroblewska-Seniuk KE, Dabrowski P, Szyfter W, Mazela J. Universal newborn hearing screening: Methods and results, obstacles, and benefits. *Pediatr Res* 2017;81(3):415–22.
16. Merten S, Dratva J, Ackermann-Liebrich U. Do baby-friendly hospitals influence breastfeeding duration on a national level? *Pediatrics* 2005;116(5):e702–8.
17. Jaafar SH, Ho JJ, Lee KS. Rooming-in for new mother and infant versus separate care for increasing the duration of breastfeeding. *Cochrane Database Syst Rev* 2016;(8):CD006641.
18. Lipke B, Gilbert G, Shimer H, et al. Newborn safety bundle to prevent falls and promote safe sleep. *MCN Am J Matern Child Nurs* 2018;43(1):32–37.
19. Thach BT. Deaths and near deaths of healthy newborn infants while bed sharing on maternity wards. *J Perinatol* 2014;34(4):275–79.
20. Lipke B et al. Newborn safety bundle to prevent falls.

21. Flaherman VJ, Schaefer EW, Kuzniewicz MW, Li SX, Walsh EM, Paul IM. Early weight loss nomograms for exclusively breastfed newborns. *Pediatrics* 2015;135(1):e16–23.

22. Smith HA, Becker GE. Early additional food and fluids for healthy breastfed full-term infants. *Cochrane Database Syst Rev* 2016;(8):CD006462.

23. Committee on Hyperbilirubinemia. Management of hyperbilirubinemia in the newborn infant 35 or more weeks of gestation. *Pediatrics* 2004;114(1):297–316.

24. Chapman J, Marfurt S, Reid J. Effectiveness of delayed cord clamping in reducing postdelivery complications in preterm infants: A systematic review. *J Perinat Neonatal Nurs* 2016;30(4): 372–78.

25. McDonald SJ, Middleton P, Dowswell T, Morris PS. Effect of timing of umbilical cord clamping of term infants on maternal and neonatal outcomes. *Cochrane Database Syst Rev* 2013;(7): CD004074.

26. American Academy of Pediatrics Committee on Fetus and Newborn. Controversies concerning vitamin K and the newborn. *Pediatrics* 2003;112(1 Pt 1):191–92.

27. American Academy of Pediatrics Committee on Fetus and Newborn. Controversies concering vitamin K.

CHAPTER 2: WAIT, YOU WANT ME TO TAKE IT HOME?

1. Sun KK, Choi KY, Chow YY. Injury by mittens in neonates: A report of an unusual presentation of this easily overlooked problem and literature review. *Pediatr Emerg Care* 2007;23(10):731–34.

2. Gerard CM, Harris KA, Thach BT. Spontaneous arousals in supine infants while swaddled and unswaddled during rapid eye movement and quiet sleep. *Pediatrics* 2002;110(6):e70.

3. Van Sleuwen BE, Engelberts AC, Boere-Boonekamp MM, Kuis W, Schulpen TW, L'hoir MP. Swaddling: A systematic review. *Pediatrics* 2007;120(4):e1097–106.

4. Ohgi S, Akiyama T, Arisawa K, Shigemori K. Randomised controlled trial of swaddling versus massage in the management of excessive crying in infants with cerebral injuries. *Arch Dis Child* 2004;89(3):212–26.

5. Short MA, Brooks-Brunn JA, Reeves DS, Yeager J, Thorpe JA. The effects of swaddling versus standard positioning on neuromuscular development in very low birth weight infants. *Neonatal Netw* 1996;15(4):25–31.

6. Short MA et al. The effects of swaddling versus standard positioning.

7. Reijneveld SA, Brugman E, Hirasing RA. Excessive infant crying: The impact of varying definitions. *Pediatrics* 2001;108(4):893–97.

8. Biagioli E, Tarasco V, Lingua C, Moja L, Savino F. Pain-relieving agents for infantile colic. *Cochrane Database Syst Rev* 2016;9:CD009999.

9. Sung V, Collett S, De Gooyer T, Hiscock H, Tang M, Wake M. Probiotics to prevent or treat excessive infant crying: Systematic review and meta-analysis. *JAMA Pediatr* 2013;167(12):1150–57.

10. Iacovou M, Ralston RA, Muir J, Walker KZ, Truby H. Dietary management of infantile colic: A systematic review. *Matern Child Health J* 2012;16(6):1319–31.

11. Hill DJ, Hudson IL, Sheffield LJ, Shelton MJ, Menahem S, Hosking CS. A low allergen diet is a significant intervention in infantile colic: Results of a community-based study. *J Allergy Clin Immunol* 1995;96(6 Pt 1):886–92. Iacovou M et al. Dietary management of infantile colic.

12. Hill DJ et al. A low allergen diet is a significant intervention in infantile colic.

13. Available at https://en.wikipedia.org/wiki/Hygiene_hypothesis.

14. Hui C, Neto G, Tsertsvadze A, et al. Diagnosis and management of febrile infants (0–3 months). *Evid Rep Technol Assess (Full Rep)* 2012;(205):1–297. Maniaci V, Dauber A, Weiss S, Nylen E, Becker KL, Bachur R. Procalcitonin in young febrile infants for the detection of serious bacterial infections. *Pediatrics* 2008;122(4):701–10. Kadish HA, Loveridge B, Tobey J, Bolte RG, Corneli HM. Applying outpatient protocols in febrile infants 1–28 days of age: Can the threshold be lowered? *Clin Pediatr (Phila)* 2000;39(2):81–88. Baker MD, Bell LM. Unpredictability of serious bacterial illness in febrile infants from birth to 1 month of age. *Arch Pediatr Adolesc Med* 1999;153(5):508–11. Bachur RG, Harper MB. Predictive model for serious bacterial infections among infants younger than 3 months of age. *Pediatrics* 2001;108(2):311–16.

15. Chua KP, Neuman MI, McWilliams JM, Aronson PL. Association between clinical outcomes and hospital guidelines for cerebrospinal fluid testing in febrile infants aged 29–56 days. *J Pediatr* 2015;167(6):1340–46.e9.

CHAPTER 3: TRUST ME, TAKE THE MESH UNDERWEAR

1. Frigerio M, Manodoro S, Bernasconi DP, Verri D, Milani R, Vergani P. Incidence and risk factors of third- and fourth-degree perineal tears in a single Italian scenario. *Eur J Obstet Gynecol Reprod Biol* 2017;221:139–43. Bodner-Adler B, Bodner K, Kaider A, et al. Risk factors for third-degree perineal tears in vaginal delivery, with an analysis of episiotomy types. *J Reprod Med* 2001;46(8): 752–56. Ramm O, Woo VG, Hung YY, Chen HC, Ritterman Weintraub ML. Risk factors for the development of obstetric anal sphincter injuries in modern obstetric practice. *Obstet Gynecol* 2018;131(2):290–96.
2. Berens P. Overview of the postpartum period: Physiology, complications, and maternal care. *UpTo-Date*. Accessed 2017. Available at https://www.uptodate.com/contents/overview-of-the-postpar tum-period-physiology-complications-and-maternal-care.
3. Raul A. Exercise during pregnancy and the postpartum period. *UpToDate*. Accessed 2017. Available at https://www.uptodate.com/contents/exercise-during-pregnancy-and-the-postpartum-period.
4. Jawed-Wessel S, Sevick E. The impact of pregnancy and childbirth on sexual behaviors: A systematic review. *J Sex Res* 2017;54(4–5):411–23. Lurie S, Aizenberg M, Sulema V, et al. Sexual function after childbirth by the mode of delivery: A prospective study. *Arch Gynecol Obstet* 2013;288(4): 785–92.
5. Viguera A. Postpartum unipolar major depression: Epidemiology, clinical features, assessment, and diagnosis. *UpToDate*. Accessed 2017. Available at https://www.uptodate.com/contents/postpar tum-unipolar-major-depression-epidemiology-clinical-features-assessment-and-diagnosis.
6. O'Connor E, Rossom RC, Henninger M, Groom HC, Burda BU. Primary care screening for and treat-ment of depression in pregnant and postpartum women: Evidence report and systematic review for the US Preventive Services Task Force. *JAMA* 2016;315(4):388–406.
7. Payne J. Postpartum psychosis: Epidemiology, pathogenesis, clinical manifestations, course, assess-ment, and diagnosis. *UpToDate*. Accessed 2017. Available at https://www.uptodate.com/contents /postpartum-psychosis-epidemiology-pathogenesis-clinical-manifestations-course-assessment -and-diagnosis.

CHAPTER 4: BREAST IS BEST? BREAST IS BETTER? BREAST IS ABOUT THE SAME?

1. La Leche League International. Available at http://www.llli.org/resources. Fit Pregnancy and Baby. *Fit Pregnancy and Baby—Prenatal & Postnatal Guidance on Health, Exercise, Baby Care, Sex & More.* https://www.fitpregnancy.com, https://www.fitpregnancy.com/baby/breastfeeding/20 -breastfeeding-benefits-mom-baby.
2. Fomon S. Infant feeding in the 20th century: Formula and beikost. *J Nutr* 2001;131(2):409S–20S.
3. Angelsen N, Vik T, Jacobsen G, Bakketeig L. Breast feeding and cognitive development at age 1 and 5 years. *Arch Dis Child* 2001;85(3):183–88.
4. Der G, Batty GD, Deary IJ. Effect of breast feeding on intelligence in children: Prospective study, sibling pairs analysis, and meta-analysis. *BMJ* 2006;333(7575):945.
5. Der G et al. Effect of breast feeding on intelligence in children.
6. Kramer MS, Chalmers B, Hodnett ED, Sevkovskaya Z, Dzikovich I, Shapiro S, Collet J, Vanilovich I, Mezen I, Ducruet T, Shishko G, Zubovich V, Mknuik D, Gluchanina E, Dombrovskiy V, Ustinovitch A, Kot T, Bogdanovich N, Ovchinikova L, Helsing E, for the PROBIT Study Group. Promotion of Breastfeeding Intervention Trial (PROBIT): A randomized trial in the Republic of Belarus. *JAMA* 2001;285(4):413–20.
7. Kramer MS et al. PROBIT.
8. For the statistically minded, simply scaling by multiplying to make the effect bigger is not that straightforward and requires further assumptions about the nature of the treatment, so it is com-mon to simply report these effects as what we call "intent to treat" or just the difference between the treatment and the control groups.
9. Quigley M, McGuire W. Formula versus donor breast milk for feeding preterm or low birth weight infants. *Cochrane Database Syst Rev* 2014;(4):CD002971.
10. Bowatte G, Tham R, Allen K, Tan D, Lau M, Dai X, Lodge C. Breastfeeding and childhood acute otitis media: A systematic review and meta-analysis. *Acta Paediatr* 2015;104(467):85–95.
11. Kørvel-Hanquist A, Koch A, Niclasen J, et al. Risk factors of early otitis media in the Danish Na-tional Birth Cohort. Torrens C, ed. *PLoS ONE* 2016;11(11):e0166465.

12. Quigley MA, Carson C, Sacker A, Kelly Y. Exclusive breastfeeding duration and infant infection. *Eur J Clin Nutr* 2016;70(12):1420–27.

13. Carpenter R, McGarvey C, Mitchell EA, et al. Bed sharing when parents do not smoke: Is there a risk of SIDS? An individual level analysis of five major case-control studies. *BMJ Open* 2013;3:e002299.

14. Hauck FR, Thompson JMD, Tanabe KO, Moon RY, Mechtild MV. Breastfeeding and reduced risk of sudden infant death syndrome: A meta-analysis. *Pediatrics* 2011;128(1):103–10.

15. Thompson JMD, Tanabe K, Moon RY, et al. Duration of breastfeeding and risk of SIDS: An individual participant data meta-analysis. *Pediatrics* 2017;140(5).

16. Vennemann MM, Bajanowski T, Brinkmann B, Jorch G, Yücesan K, Sauerland C, Mitchell EA. Does breastfeeding reduce the risk of sudden infant death syndrome? *Pediatrics* 2009;123(3):e406–e410.

17. Fleming PJ, Blair PS, Bacon C, et al. Environment of infants during sleep and risk of the sudden infant death syndrome: Results of 1993–5 case-control study for confidential inquiry into stillbirths and deaths in infancy. Confidential enquiry into stillbirths and deaths regional coordinators and researchers. *BMJ* 1996;313(7051):191–95.

18. Kramer MS et al. PROBIT.

19. Martin RM, Patel R, Kramer MS, et al. Effects of promoting longer-term and exclusive breastfeeding on cardiometabolic risk factors at age 11.5 years: A cluster-randomized, controlled trial. *Circulation* 2014;129(3):321–29.

20. Colen CG, Ramey DM. Is breast truly best? Estimating the effects of breastfeeding on long-term child health and wellbeing in the United States using sibling comparisons. *Soc Sci Med* 2014;109: 55–65. Nelson MC, Gordon-Larsen P, Adair LS. Are adolescents who were breast-fed less likely to be overweight? Analyses of sibling pairs to reduce confounding. *Epidemiology* 2005;16(2):247–53.

21. Owen CG, Martin RM, Whincup PH, Davey-Smith G, Gillman MW, Cook DG. The effect of breastfeeding on mean body mass index throughout life: A quantitative review of published and unpublished observational evidence. *Am J Clin Nutr* 2005;82(6):1298–307.

22. Kindgren E, Fredrikson M, Ludvigsson J. Early feeding and risk of juvenile idiopathic arthritis: A case control study in a prospective birth cohort. *Pediatr Rheumatol Online J* 2017;15:46. Rosenberg AM. Evaluation of associations between breast feeding and subsequent development of juvenile rheumatoid arthritis. *J Rheumatol* 1996;23(6):1080–82. Silfverdal SA, Bodin L, Olcén P. Protective effect of breastfeeding: An ecologic study of Haemophilus influenzae meningitis and breastfeeding in a Swedish population. *Int J Epidemiol* 1999;28(1):152–56. Lamberti LM, Zakarija-Grkovi I, Fischer Walker CL, et al. Breastfeeding for reducing the risk of pneumonia morbidity and mortality in children under two: A systematic literature review and meta-analysis. *BMC Public Health* 2013;13(Suppl 3):S18. Li R, Dee D, Li C-M, Hoffman HJ, Grummer-Strawn LM. Breastfeeding and risk of infections at 6 years. *Pediatrics* 2014;134(Suppl 1):S13–S20. Niewiadomski O, Studd C, Wilson J, et al. Influence of food and lifestyle on the risk of developing inflammatory bowel disease. *Intern Med J* 2016;46(6):669–76. Hansen TS, Jess T, Vind I, et al. Environmental factors in inflammatory bowel disease: A case-control study based on a Danish inception cohort. *J Crohns Colitis* 2011;5(6):577–84.

23. Type 1 diabetes, also known as juvenile diabetes, is the type that develops in childhood and requires insulin injections. In 2017 researchers in northern Europe using a rich trove of data from two countries published a paper arguing that babies who are not breastfed are more likely to develop this disease (Lund-Blix NA, Dydensborg Sander S, Størdal K, et al. Infant feeding and risk of type 1 diabetes in two large Scandinavian birth cohorts. *Diabetes Care* 2017;40[7]:920–27). This study was motivated by a set of small case-control studies that showed similar effects (see references in this paper). To be more precise, the authors showed that the babies of mothers who *never try to breastfeed at all* are more likely to develop type 1 diabetes than those who breastfeed even a bit.

I am skeptical of these conclusions, despite the quality of the data and large sample size. The main issue is that in this population, not breastfeeding at all is very unusual—only 1 to 2 percent of women make this choice. These women differ in many ways from those who breastfed (including being more likely to be diabetic themselves), and even with good data we cannot hope to see all these ways. When a choice is so unusual, we really worry about what drives it.

The researchers' conclusions may be correct, but we simply need more data (ideally from a setting where not breastfeeding at all is more common) to be confident.

Leukemia is the most common type of childhood cancer, and it has been hypothesized that it is linked to not breastfeeding. Like SIDS, this is rare, and researchers studying it typically use a case-control design: recruiting families with children with leukemia and a comparison group of children without a cancer diagnosis. In 2015 a large review article combined a number of small studies of this, and argued that together they show a significant reduction in the risk of cancer for children who are breastfed (Amitay EL, Keinan-Boker L. Breastfeeding and childhood leukemia incidence: A meta-analysis and systematic review. *JAMA Pediatr* 2015;169[6]:e151025).

However, as other authors note, this conclusion is fragile (Ojha RP, Asdahl PH. Breastfeeding and childhood leukemia incidence duplicate data inadvertently included in the meta-analysis and consideration of possible confounders. *JAMA Pediatr* 2015;169[11]:1070). In the main analysis—the one on which the primary conclusions are based—researchers do not take into account any other differences between the children with leukemia and those without besides the cancer diagnosis. But many other factors differ across the two groups. Taking into account even just the differences in the ages of the mothers makes the effects much smaller and not statistically significant. The effect may well be even less compelling if we adjusted for more differences.

24. Der G, Batty GD, Deary IJ. Effect of breast feeding on intelligence in children: Prospective study, sibling pairs analysis, and meta-analysis. *BMJ* 2006;333(7575):945.
25. Specifically, when they look at the results from independent evaluators, they do not see differences in verbal IQ. These show up only in the evaluations done by the study personnel. This difference suggests evaluator bias.
26. Der G, Batty GD, Deary IJ. Results from the PROBIT breastfeeding trial may have been overinterpreted. *Arch Gen Psychiatry* 2008;65(12):1456–57.
27. Krause KM, Lovelady CA, Peterson BL, Chowdhury N, Østbye T. Effect of breast-feeding on weight retention at 3 and 6 months postpartum: Data from the North Carolina WIC Programme. *Public Health Nutr* 2010;13(12):2019–26.
28. Woolhouse H, James J, Gartland D, McDonald E, Brown SJ. Maternal depressive symptoms at three months postpartum and breastfeeding rates at six months postpartum: Implications for primary care in a prospective cohort study of primiparous women in Australia. *Women Birth* 2016;29(4): 381–87.
29. Crandall CJ, Liu J, Cauley J, et al. Associations of parity, breastfeeding, and fractures in the Women's Health Observational Study. *Obstet Gynecol* 2017;130(1):171–80.

CHAPTER 5: BREASTFEEDING: A HOW-TO GUIDE

1. Sharma A. Efficacy of early skin-to-skin contact on the rate of exclusive breastfeeding in term neonates: A randomized controlled trial. *Afr Health Sci* 2016;16(3):790–97.
2. Moore ER, Bergman N, Anderson GC, Medley N. Early skin-to-skin contact for mothers and their healthy newborn infants. *Cochrane Database Syst Rev* 2016;11:CD003519.
3. Balogun OO, O'Sullivan EJ, McFadden A, et al. Interventions for promoting the initiation of breastfeeding. *Cochrane Database Syst Rev* 2016;11:CD001688.
4. McKeever P, Stevens B, Miller KL, et al. Home versus hospital breastfeeding support for newborns: A randomized controlled trial. *Birth* 2002;29(4):258–65.
5. Jaafar SH, Ho JJ, Lee KS. Rooming-in for new mother and infant versus separate care for increasing the duration of breastfeeding. *Cochrane Database Syst Rev* 2016;(8):CD006641.
6. Chow S, Chow R, Popovic M, et al. The use of nipple shields: A review. *Front Public Health* 2015;3:236.
7. Meier PP, Brown LP, Hurst NM, et al. Nipple shields for preterm infants: Effect on milk transfer and duration of breastfeeding. *J Hum Lact* 2000;16(2):106–14.
8. Meier PP et al. Nipple shields for preterm infants.
9. Walsh J, Tunkel D. Diagnosis and treatment of ankyloglossia in newborns and infants: A review. *JAMA Otolaryngol Head Neck Surg* 2017;143(10):1032–39.
10. O'Shea JE, Foster JP, O'Donnell CP, et al. Frenotomy for tongue-tie in newborn infants. *Cochrane Database Syst Rev* 2017;3:CD011065.
11. Dennis CL, Jackson K, Watson J. Interventions for treating painful nipples among breastfeeding women. *Cochrane Database Syst Rev* 2014;(12):CD007366.
12. Mohammadzadeh A, Farhat A, Esmaeily H. The effect of breast milk and lanolin on sore nipples. *Saudi Med J* 2005;26(8):1231–34.
13. Dennis CL et al. Interventions for treating painful nipples.
14. Jaafar SH, Ho JJ, Jahanfar S, Angolkar M. Effect of restricted pacifier use in breastfeeding term infants for increasing duration of breastfeeding. *Cochrane Database Syst Rev* 2016;(8):CD007202.
15. Kramer MS, Barr RG, Dagenais S, Yang H, Jones P, Ciofani L, Jané F. Pacifier use, early weaning, and cry/fuss behavior: A randomized controlled trial. *JAMA* 2001;286(3):322–26.

16. Howard CR, Howard FR, Lanphear B, Eberly S, DeBlieck EA, Oakes D, Lawrence RA. Randomized clinical trial of pacifier use and bottle-feeding or cupfeeding and their effect on breastfeeding. *Pediatrics* 2003;111(3):511–18.

17. This study also evaluates pacifier use on breastfeeding. For most outcomes and specifications, it found no impact of early pacifier use on breastfeeding success; for one specification researchers found some significant effects, although these effects are small and do not survive an adjustment for the multiple hypothesis testing.

18. Brownell E, Howard CR, Lawrence RA, Dozier AM. Delayed onset lactogenesis II predicts the cessation of any or exclusive breastfeeding. *J Pediatr* 2012;161(4):608–14.

19. Brownell E et al. Delayed onset lactogenesis II.

20. Brownell E et al. Delayed onset lactogenesis II. Garcia AH, Voortman T, Baena CP, et al. Maternal weight status, diet, and supplement use as determinants of breastfeeding and complementary feeding: A systematic review and meta-analysis. *Nutr Rev* 2016;74(8):490–516. Zhu P, Hao J, Jiang X, Huang K, Tao F. New insight into onset of lactation: Mediating the negative effect of multiple perinatal biopsychosocial stress on breastfeeding duration. *Breastfeed Med* 2013;8:151–58.

21. Ndikom CM, Fawole B, Ilesanmi RE. Extra fluids for breastfeeding mothers for increasing milk production. *Cochrane Database Syst Rev* 2014;(6):CD008758.

22. Bazzano AN, Hofer R, Thibeau S, Gillispie V, Jacobs M, Theall KP. A review of herbal and pharmaceutical galactagogues for breast-feeding. *Ochsner J* 2016;16(4):511–24.

23. Bazzano AN et al. A review of herbal and pharmaceutical galactagogues for breast-feeding. Donovan TJ, Buchanan K. Medications for increasing milk supply in mothers expressing breastmilk for their preterm hospitalised infants. *Cochrane Database Syst Rev* 2012;(3):CD005544.

24. Spencer J. Common problems of breastfeeding and weaning. *UpToDate.* Accessed 2017. Available at https://www.uptodate.com/contents/common-problems-of-breastfeeding-and-weaning.

25. Mangesi L, Zakarija-Grkovic I. Treatments for breast engorgement during lactation. *Cochrane Database Syst Rev* 2016;(6):CD006946.

26. Butte N, Stuebe A. Maternal nutrition during lactation. *UpToDate.* Accessed 2018. Available at https://www.uptodate.com/contents/maternal-nutrition-during-lactation.

27. Lust KD, Brown J, Thomas W. Maternal intake of cruciferous vegetables and other foods and colic symptoms in exclusively breast-fed infants. *J Acad Nutr Diet* 1996;96(1):46–48.

28. Haastrup MB, Pottegård A, Damkier P. Alcohol and breastfeeding. *Basic Clin Pharmacol Toxicol* 2014;114(2):168–73.

29. Haastrup MB et al. Alcohol and breastfeeding.

30. https://www.beststart.org/resources/alc_reduction/pdf/brstfd_alc_deskref_eng.pdf.

31. Haastrup MB et al. Alcohol and breastfeeding.

32. Be Safe: Have an Alcohol Free Pregnancy. Revised 2012. https://www.toxnet.nlm.nih.gov/new toxnet/lactmed.htm.

33. Lazaryan M, Shasha Zigelman C, Dagan Z, Berkovitch M. Codeine should not be prescribed for breastfeeding mothers or children under the age of 12. *Acta paediatrica* 2015;104(6):550–56.

34. Lam J, Kelly L, Ciszkowski C, Landsmeer ML, Nauta M, Carleton BC, et al. Central nervous system depression of neonates breastfed by mothers receiving oxycodone for postpartum analgesia. *J Pediatr* 2012;160(1):33–37.

35. Kimmel M, Meltzer-Brody S. Safety of infant exposure to antidepressants and benzodiazepines through breastfeeding. *UpToDate.* Accessed 2018. Available at https://www.uptodate.com/con tents/safety-of-infant-exposure-to-antidepressants-and-benzodiazepines-through-breastfeeding.

36. Acuña-Muga J, Ureta-Velasco N, De la Cruz-Bértolo J, et al. Volume of milk obtained in relation to location and circumstances of expression in mothers of very low birth weight infants. *J Hum Lact* 2014;30(1):41–46.

CHAPTER 6: SLEEP POSITION AND LOCATION

1. Horne RS, Ferens D, Watts AM, et al. The prone sleeping position impairs arousability in term infants. *J Pediatr* 2001;138(6):811–16.

2. Dwyer T, Ponsonby AL. Sudden infant death syndrome and prone sleeping position. *Ann Epidemiol* 2009;19(4):245–49.

3. Spock B, Rothenberg M. *Dr. Spock's Baby and Child Care.* New York: Simon and Schuster, 1977.

4. There is a good example in a study from the 1990s (Dwyer T, Ponsonby AL, Newman NM, Gibbons LE. Prospective cohort study of prone sleeping position and sudden infant death syndrome. *Lancet*

1991; 337[8752]:1244–47). In this study, researchers attempted to follow a cohort over time and study what determines SIDS deaths. They enrolled 3,110 people, and in that population, there were 23 SIDS deaths. The researchers were able to obtain information on sleep position for 15 of these deaths, which wasn't enough to draw statistical conclusions.

5. Fleming PJ, Gilbert R, Azaz Y, et al. Interaction between bedding and sleeping position in the sudden infant death syndrome: A population based case-control study. *BMJ* 1990;301(6743):85–89.

6. Ponsonby AL, Dwyer T, Gibbons LE, Cochrane JA, Wang YG. Factors potentiating the risk of sudden infant death syndrome associated with the prone position. *N Engl J Med* 1993;329(6):377–82. Dwyer T et al. Prospective cohort study of prone sleeping position.

7. Engelberts AC, De Jonge GA, Kostense PJ. An analysis of trends in the incidence of sudden infant death in the Netherlands 1969–89. *J Paediatr Child Health* 1991;27(6):329–33.

8. Guntheroth WG, Spiers PS. Sleeping prone and the risk of sudden infant death syndrome. *JAMA* 1992;267(17):2359–62.

9. Willinger M, Hoffman HJ, Wu K, Hou J, Kessler RC, Ward SL, Keens TG, Corwin MJ. Factors associated with the transition to nonprone sleep positions of infants in the United States: The National Infant Sleep Position Study. *JAMA* 1998;280(4):329–35.

10. Branch LG, Kesty K, Krebs E, Wright L, Leger S, David LR. Deformational plagiocephaly and craniosynostosis: Trends in diagnosis and treatment after the "Back to Sleep" campaign. *J Craniofac Surg* 2015;26(1):147–50. Peitsch WK, Keefer CH, Labrie RA, Mulliken JB. Incidence of cranial asymmetry in healthy newborns. *Pediatrics* 2002;110(6):e72.

11. Peitsch WK et al. Incidence of cranial asymmetry in healthy newborns. *Pediatrics* 2002;110(6):e72.

12. Van Wijk RM, Van Vlimmeren LA, Groothuis-Oudshoorn CG, Van der Ploeg CP, Ijzerman MJ, Boere-Boonekamp MM. Helmet therapy in infants with positional skull deformation: Randomised controlled trial. *BMJ* 2014;348:g2741.

13. Carpenter R et al. Bed sharing when parents do not smoke.

14. Vennemann MM, Hense HW, Bajanowski T, et al. Bed sharing and the risk of sudden infant death syndrome: Can we resolve the debate? *J Pediatr* 2012;160(1):44–48.e2.

15. CDC Fact Sheets, "Health Effects of Secondhand Smoke." Updated January 2017. https://www.cdc.gov/tobacco/data_statistics/fact_sheets/secondhand_smoke/health_effects/index.htm.

16. Scragg R, Mitchell EA, Taylor BJ, et al. Bed sharing, smoking, and alcohol in the sudden infant death syndrome. New Zealand Cot Death Study Group. *BMJ* 1993;307(6915):1312–18.

17. Horsley T, Clifford T, Barrowman N, Bennett S, Yazdi F, Sampson M, Moher D, Dingwall O, Schachter H, Côté A. Benefits and harms associated with the practice of bed sharing: A systematic review. *Arch Pediatr Adolesc Med* 2007;161(3):237–45. doi:10.1001/archpedi.161.3.237.

18. Ball HL, Howel D, Bryant A, Best E, Russell C, Ward-Platt M. Bed-sharing by breastfeeding mothers: Who bed-shares and what is the relationship with breastfeeding duration?. *Acta Paediatr* 2016;105(6):628–34.

19. Ball HL, Ward-Platt MP, Howel D, Russell C. Randomised trial of sidecar crib use on breastfeeding duration (NECOT). *Arch Dis Child* 2011;96(7):630–34.

20. Blair PS, Fleming PJ, Smith IJ, et al. Babies sleeping with parents: Case-control study of factors influencing the risk of the sudden infant death syndrome. *BMJ* 1999;319(7223):1457–62.

21. Carpenter RG, Irgens LM, Blair PS, et al. Sudden unexplained infant death in 20 regions in Europe: Case control study. *Lancet* 2004;363(9404):185–91.

22. Tappin D, Ecob R, Brooke H. Bedsharing, roomsharing, and sudden infant death syndrome in Scotland: A case-control study. *J Pediatr* 2005;147(1):32–37. Scragg RK, Mitchell EA, Stewart AW, et al. Infant room-sharing and prone sleep position in sudden infant death syndrome. New Zealand Cot Death Study Group. *Lancet* 1996;347(8993):7–12.

23. Tappin D et al. Bedsharing, roomsharing, and sudden infant death syndrome in Scotland.

24. Tappin D et al. Bedsharing, roomsharing, and sudden infant death syndrome in Scotland. Carpenter RG et al. Sudden unexplained infant death in 20 regions in Europe.

25. Scheers NJ, Woodard DW, Thach BT. Crib bumpers continue to cause infant deaths: A need for a new preventive approach. *J Pediatr* 2016;169:93–97.e1.

CHAPTER 7: ORGANIZE YOUR BABY

1. Weissbluth M. *Healthy Sleep Habits, Happy Child.* New York: Ballantine Books, 2015.

2. Galland BC, Taylor BJ, Elder DE, Herbison P. Normal sleep patterns in infants and children: A systematic review of observational studies. *Sleep Med Rev* 2012;16(3):213–22.

3. Mindell JA, Leichman ES, Composto J, Lee C, Bhullar B, Walters RM. Development of infant and toddler sleep patterns: Real-world data from a mobile application. *J Sleep Res* 2016;25(5):508–16.

CHAPTER 8: VACCINATION: YES, PLEASE

1. CDC. *Measles (Rubeola)*. Available at https://www.cdc.gov/measles/about/history.html.
2. Oster E. Does disease cause vaccination? Disease outbreaks and vaccination response. *J Health Econ* 2017;57:90–101.
3. The story of Wakefield and his impact on vaccine rates is told in much more detail in Seth Mnookin's wonderful book *Panic Virus*. New York: Simon & Schuster, 2012. Brian Deer also has an excellent set of articles summarizing the issues in the *British Medical Journal* (Deer B. Secrets of the MMR scare: How the vaccine crisis was meant to make money. *BMJ* 2011;342:c5258).
4. Wakefield AJ, Murch SH, Anthony A, Linnell J, Casson DM, Malik M, Berelowitz M, Dhillon AP, Thomson MA, Harvey P, Valentine A, Davies SE, Walker-Smith JA. Retracted: Ileal-lymphoid-nodular hyperplasia, non-specific colitis, and pervasive developmental disorder in children. *Lancet* 1998;351(9103):637–41.
5. Committee to Review Adverse Effects of Vaccines. Adverse effects of vaccines: Evidence and causality. National Academies Press, 2012.
6. The report includes the flu vaccine, but many of those links focus on adults, and I will focus here on childhood vaccinations.
7. Verity CM, Butler NR, Golding J. Febrile convulsions in a national cohort followed up from birth. I—Prevalence and recurrence in the first five years of life. *Br Med J (Clin Res Ed)* 1985;290(6478): 1307–10.
8. Chen RT, Glasser JW, Rhodes PH, et al. Vaccine Safety Datalink project: A new tool for improving vaccine safety monitoring in the United States. The Vaccine Safety Datalink Team. *Pediatrics* 1997;99(6):765–73.
9. Madsen KM, Hviid A, Vestergaard M, et al. A population-based study of measles, mumps, and rubella vaccination and autism. *N Engl J Med* 2002;347(19):1477–82.
10. Jain A, Marshall J, Buikema A, Bancroft T, Kelly JP, Newschaffer CJ. Autism occurrence by MMR vaccine status among US children with older siblings with and without autism. *JAMA* 2015;313(15): 1534–40.
11. Gadad BS, Li W, Yazdani U, et al. Administration of thimerosal-containing vaccines to infant rhesus macaques does not result in autism-like behavior or neuropathology. *Proc Natl Acad Sci USA* 2015;112(40):12498–503.
12. Occasionally, an academic paper will come out that will restate this claim. An example is one published in 2014 in the journal *Translational Neurodegeneration* (Hooker BS. Measles-mumps-rubella vaccination timing and autism among young African American boys: A reanalysis of CDC data. *Transl Neurodegener* 2014;3:16). The author of this paper uses a small sample of children and a case-control design—taking some kids with autism and matching them to some children without autism. He argues that for African American boys in particular the risk of autism is higher if they get the MMR vaccine before 36 months.

   This paper is an almost comically bad example of how to do statistics. The author finds no effect overall, so he moves to looking for effects in little groups. This is not an approved way to do research—even if there is truly no relationship, you'll almost always be able to find some small group where there is an effect, just by chance. It turns out the relationship is robust only for African American boys who are low birth weight, and only when the author considers vaccinations before 36 months, not before 18 months or 24 months. There is no information on sample size reported (also a no-no in paper writing), but it seems like some of these relationships are based on 5 or 10 children total.

   Moreover, the author of this paper—Brian Hooker—is a well-known antivaccination advocate who, like Wakefield, has an interest in promoting the antivaccination viewpoint since it benefits his expert litigation practice. This information was not fully disclosed in the article, as it should have been, and because of this conflict and the statistical problems, this paper was retracted, just like the Wakefield paper, but, of course, not before it got a lot of coverage and scaremongering in the media. It is unfortunate that there is not more interest in covering the many well-conducted and large studies that show this relationship is complete bunk.
13. Omer SB, Pan WKY, Halsey NA, Stokley S, Moulton LH, Navar AM, Pierce M, Salmon DA. Non-medical exemptions to school immunization requirements: Secular trends and association of state policies with pertussis incidence. *JAMA* 2006;296(14):1757–63.

14. Verity CM et al. Febrile convulsions in a national cohort followed up from birth.
15. Pesco P, Bergero P, Fabricius G, Hozbor D. Mathematical modeling of delayed pertussis vaccination in infants. *Vaccine* 2015;33(41):5475–80.

CHAPTER 9: STAY-AT-HOME MOM? STAY-AT-WORK MOM?

1. For a review, see http://web.stanford.edu/~mrossin/RossinSlater_maternity_family_leave.pdf.
2. Goldberg WA, Prause J, Lucas-Thompson R, Himsel A. Maternal employment and children's achievement in context: A meta-analysis of four decades of research. *Psychol Bull* 2008;134(1):77–108.
3. Goldberg WA et al. Maternal employment and children's achievement in context.
4. These studies also show that when you look at *changes* in test scores between years it doesn't matter what the working configuration is, suggesting that it may be underlying differences that matter.
5. Ruhm CJ. Maternal employment and adolescent development. *Labour Econ* 2008;15(5):958–83.
6. Marantz S, Mansfield A. Maternal employment and the development of sex-role stereotyping in five-to eleven-year-old girls. *Child Dev* 1997;48(2):668–73. McGinn KL, Castro MR, Lingo EL. Mums the word! Cross-national effects of maternal employment on gender inequalities at work and at home. *Harvard Business School* 2015;15(194).
7. Rossin-Slater M. The effects of maternity leave on children's birth and infant health outcomes in the United States. *J Health Econ* 2011;30(2):221–39.
8. Rossin-Slater M. Maternity and Family Leave Policy. *Natl Bureau Econ Res* 2017.
9. Rossin-Slater M. Maternity and Family Leave Policy.
10. Carneiro P, Loken KV, Kjell GS. A flying start? Maternity leave benefits and long-run outcomes of children. *J Pol Econ* 2015;123(2):365–412.
11. This is an approximate calculation based on a medium-tax-level state.

CHAPTER 10: WHO SHOULD TAKE CARE OF THE BABY?

1. NICHD Early Childcare Research Network. Early childcare and children's development prior to school entry: Results from the NICHD Study of Early Childcare. *AERJ* 2002;39(1):133–64.
2. Belsky J, Vandell DL, Burchinal M, et al. Are there long-term effects of early childcare?. *Child Dev* 2007;78(2):681–701.
3. NICHD. Type of childcare and children's development at 54 months. *Early Childhood Res Q* 2004;19(2):203–30.
4. NICHD. Early childcare and children's development prior to school entry.
5. Belsky J et al. Are there long-term effects of early childcare?
6. Broberg AG, Wessels H, Lamb ME, Hwang CP. Effects of day care on the development of cognitive abilities in 8-year-olds: A longitudinal study. *Dev Psychol* 1997;33(1):62–69.
7. Huston AC, Bobbitt KC, Bentley A. Time spent in childcare: How and why does it affect social development? *Dev Psychol* 2015;51(5):621–34.
8. NICHD. The effects of infant childcare on infant-mother attachment security: Results of the NICHD Study of Early Childcare. *Child Dev* 1997;68(5):860–79.
9. Augustine JM, Crosnoe RL, Gordon R. Early childcare and illness among preschoolers. *J Health Soc Behav* 2013;54(3):315–34. Enserink R, Lugnér A, Suijkerbuijk A, Bruijning-Verhagen P, Smit HA, Van Pelt W. Gastrointestinal and respiratory illness in children that do and do not attend child day care centers: A cost-of-illness study. *PLoS ONE* 2014;9(8):e104940. Morrissey TW. Multiple childcare arrangements and common communicable illnesses in children aged 3 to 54 months. *Matern Child Health J* 2013;17(7):1175–84. Bradley RH, Vandell DL. Childcare and the well-being of children. *Arch Pediatr Adolesc Med* 2007;161(7):669–76.
10. Ball TM, Holberg CJ, Aldous MB, Martinez FD, Wright AL. Influence of attendance at day care on the common cold from birth through 13 years of age. *Arch Pediatr Adolesc Med* 2002;156(2):121–26.

CHAPTER 11: SLEEP TRAINING

1. Ramos KD, Youngclarke DM. Parenting advice books about child sleep: Cosleeping and crying it out. *Sleep* 2006;29(12):1616–23.
2. Narvaez D. Dangers of "Crying It Out." *Psychology Today.* December 11, 2011. https://www.psychology today.com/blog/moral-landscapes/201112/dangers-crying-it-out.

3. This review overall includes more than 2,500 children across 52 studies, all employing variations on sleep training. Some of these studies are better than others, but there are at least 13 randomized controlled trials of "cry it out" programs. Mindell JA, Kuhn B, Lewin DS, Meltzer LJ, Sadeh A. Behavioral treatment of bedtime problems and night wakings in infants and young children. *Sleep* 2006;29(10):1263–76.

4. Kerr SM, Jowett SA, Smith LN. Preventing sleep problems in infants: A randomized controlled trial. *J Adv Nurs* 1996;24(5):938–42.

5. Hiscock H, Bayer J, Gold L, Hampton A, Ukoumunne OC, Wake M. Improving infant sleep and maternal mental health: A cluster randomised trial. *Arch Dis Child* 2007;92(11):952–58.

6. Mindell JA et al. Behavioral treatment of bedtime problems and night wakings.

7. Leeson R, Barbour J, Romaniuk D, Warr R. Management of infant sleep problems in a residential unit. *Childcare Health Dev* 1994;20(2):89–100.

8. Eckerberg, B. Treatment of sleep problems in families with young children: Effects of treatment on family well-being. *Acta Pædiatrica* 2004;93:126–34.

9. Mindell JA et al. Behavioral treatment of bedtime problems and night wakings.

10. Gradisar M, Jackson K, Spurrier NJ, et al. Behavioral interventions for infant sleep problems: A randomized controlled trial. *Pediatrics* 2016;137(6).

11. Hiscock H et al. Improving infant sleep and maternal mental health.

12. Price AM, Wake M, Ukoumunne OC, Hiscock H. Five-year follow-up of harms and benefits of behavioral infant sleep intervention: Randomized trial. *Pediatrics* 2012;130(4):643–51.

13. Blunden SL, Thompson KR, Dawson D. Behavioural sleep treatments and night time crying in infants: Challenging the status quo. *Sleep Med Rev* 2011;15(5):327–34.

14. Blunden SL et al. Behavioural sleep treatments and night time crying in infants.

15. Middlemiss W, Granger DA, Goldberg WA, Nathans L. Asynchrony of mother-infant hypothalamic-pituitary-adrenal axis activity following extinction of infant crying responses induced during the transition to sleep. *Early Hum Dev* 2012;88(4):227–32.

16. Kuhn BR, Elliott AJ. Treatment efficacy in behavioral pediatric sleep medicine. *J Psychosom Res* 2003;54(6):587–97.

CHAPTER 12: BEYOND THE BOOBS: INTRODUCING SOLID FOOD

1. Du Toit G, Katz Y, Sasieni P, et al. Early consumption of peanuts in infancy is associated with a low prevalence of peanut allergy. *J Allergy Clin Immunol* 2008;122(5):984–91.

2. Du Toit G, Roberts G, Sayre PH, et al. Randomized trial of peanut consumption in infants at risk for peanut allergy. *N Engl J Med* 2015;372(9):803–13.

3. For a discussion of updated and older guidelines, see Togias A, Cooper SF, Acebal ML, et al. Addendum guidelines for the prevention of peanut allergy in the United States: Report of the National Institute of Allergy and Infectious Diseases–sponsored expert panel. *J Allergy Clin Immunol* 2017;139(1):29–44.

4. Brown A, Jones SW, Rowan H. Baby-led weaning: The evidence to date. *Curr Nutr Rep* 2017;6(2):148–56.

5. Taylor RW, Williams SM, Fangupo LJ, et al. Effect of a baby-led approach to complementary feeding on infant growth and overweight: A randomized clinical trial. *JAMA Pediatr* 2017;171(9):838–46.

6. Moorcroft KE, Marshall JL, Mccormick FM. Association between timing of introducing solid foods and obesity in infancy and childhood: A systematic review. *Matern Child Nutr* 2011;7(1):3–26.

7. Rose CM, Birch LL, Savage JS. Dietary patterns in infancy are associated with child diet and weight outcomes at 6 years. *Int J Obes (Lond)* 2017;41(5):783–88.

8. Mennella JA, Trabulsi JC. Complementary foods and flavor experiences: Setting the foundation. *Ann Nutr Metab* 2012;60 (Suppl 2):40–50.

9. Mennella JA, Nicklaus S, Jagolino AL, Yourshaw LM. Variety is the spice of life: Strategies for promoting fruit and vegetable acceptance during infancy. *Physiol Behav* 2008;94(1):29–38. Mennella JA, Trabulsi JC. Complementary foods and flavor experiences.

10. Atkin D. The caloric costs of culture: Evidence from Indian migrants. *Amer Econ Rev* 2016;106(4):1144–81.

11. Leung AK, Marchand V, Sauve RS. The "picky eater": The toddler or preschooler who does not eat. *Paediatr Child Health* 2012;17(8):455–60.

12. Fries LR, Martin N, Van der Horst K. Parent-child mealtime interactions associated with toddlers' refusals of novel and familiar foods. *Physiol Behav* 2017;176:93–100.

13. Birch LL, Fisher JO. Development of eating behaviors among children and adolescents. *Pediatrics* 1998;101(3 Pt 2):539–49. Lafraire J, Rioux C, Giboreau A, Picard D. Food rejections in children: Cognitive and social/environmental factors involved in food neophobia and picky/fussy eating behavior. *Appetite* 2016;96:347–57.

14. Perkin MR, Logan K, Tseng A, Raji B, Ayis S, Peacock J, et al. Randomized trial of introduction of allergenic foods in breast-fed infants. *N Engl J Med* 2016;374(18):1733–43. Natsume O, Kabashima S, Nakazato J, Yamamoto-Hanada K, Narita M, Kondo M, et al. Two-step egg introduction for prevention of egg allergy in high-risk infants with eczema (PETIT): A randomised, double-blind, placebo-controlled trial. *Lancet* 2017;389(10066):276–86. Katz Y, Rajuan N, Goldberg MR, Eisenberg E, Heyman E, Cohen A, Leshno M. Early exposure to cow's milk protein is protective against IgE-mediated cow's milk protein allergy. *J Allergy Clin Immunol* 2010;126(1):77–82.

15. Hopkins D, Emmett P, Steer C, Rogers I, Noble S, Emond A. Infant feeding in the second 6 months of life related to iron status: An observational study. *Arch Dis Child* 2007;92(10):850–54.

16. Pegram PS, Stone SM. Botulism. *UpToDate*. Accessed 2017. Available at http://www.uptodate.com /contents/botulism.

17. Emmerson AJB, Dockery KE, Mughal MZ, Roberts SA, Tower CL, Berry JL. Vitamin D status of white pregnant women and infants at birth and 4 months in North West England: A cohort study. *Matern Child Nutr* 2018;14(1).

18. Greer FR, Marshall S. Bone mineral content, serum vitamin D metabolite concentrations, and ultraviolet B light exposure in infants fed human milk with and without vitamin D supplements. *J Pediatr* 1989;114(2):204–12. Naik P, Faridi MMA, Batra P, Madhu SV. Oral supplementation of parturient mothers with vitamin D and its effect on 25OHD status of exclusively breastfed infants at 6 months of age: A double-blind randomized placebo controlled trial. *Breastfeed Med* 2017;12(10):621–28.

19. Naik P et al. Oral supplementation of parturient mothers with vitamin D. Thiele DK, Ralph J, El-Masri M, Anderson CM. Vitamin D3 supplementation during pregnancy and lactation improves vitamin D status of the mother-infant dyad. *J Obstet Gynecol Neonatal Nurs* 2017;46(1):135–47.

CHAPTER 13: EARLY WALKING, LATE WALKING: PHYSICAL MILESTONES

1. Serdarevic F, Van Batenburg-Eddes T, Mous SE, et al. Relation of infant motor development with nonverbal intelligence, language comprehension and neuropsychological functioning in childhood: A population-based study. *Dev Sci* 2016;19(5):790–802.

2. Murray GK, Jones PB, Kuh D, Richards M. Infant developmental milestones and subsequent cognitive function. *Ann Neurol* 2007;62(2):128–36.

3. Much of the discussion here comes from Voigt RG. *Developmental and behavioral pediatrics*. Eds. Macias MM and Myers SM. American Academy of Pediatrics, 2011.

4. Barkoudah E, Glader L. Epidemiology, etiology and prevention of cerebral palsy. *UpToDate*. Accessed 2018. Available at https://www.uptodate.com.revproxy.brown.edu/contents/epidemiology-etiology -and-prevention-of-cerebral-palsy.

5. WHO Motor Development Study: Windows of achievement for six gross motor development milestones. *Acta Paediatr Suppl* 2006;450:86–95.

6. WHO Motor Development Study.

7. Pappas D. The common cold in children: Clinical features and diagnosis. *UpToDate*. Accessed 2018. Available at https://www.uptodate.com/contents/the-common-cold-in-children-clinical-features -and-diagnosis.

8. Pappas D. The common cold in children.

9. Klein J, Pelton S. Acute otitis media in children: Epidemiology, microbiology, clinical manifestations, and complications. *UpToDate*. Accessed 2018. Available at https://www.uptodate.com/contents /acute-otitis-media-in-children-epidemiology-microbiology-clinical-manifestations-and -complications.

CHAPTER 14: BABY EINSTEIN VS. THE TV HABIT

1. Barr R, Hayne H. Developmental changes in imitation from television during infancy. *Child Dev* 1999;70(5):1067–81.

2. Kuhl PK, Tsao FM, Liu HM. Foreign-language experience in infancy: Effects of short-term exposure and social interaction on phonetic learning. *Proc Natl Acad Sci USA* 2003;100(15):9096–101.

3. DeLoache JS, Chiong C. Babies and baby media. *Am Behav Scientist* 2009;52(8):1115–35.

4. Robb MB, Richert RA, Wartella EA. Just a talking book? Word learning from watching baby videos. *Br J Dev Psychol* 2009;27(Pt 1):27–45.

5. Richert RA, Robb MB, Fender JG, Wartella E. Word learning from baby videos. *Arch Pediatr Adolesc Med* 2010;164(5):432–37.

6. Rice ML, Woodsmall L. Lessons from television: Children's word learning when viewing. *Child Dev* 1988;59(2):420–29.

7. Bogatz GA, Ball S. *The Second Year of Sesame Street: A Continuing Evaluation*, vol. 1. Princeton, NJ: Educational Testing Service, 1971.

8. Kearney MS, Levine PB. Early childhood education by MOOC: Lessons from Sesame Street. *Natl Bureau Econ Res* working paper no. 21229, June 2016.

9. Nathanson AI, Aladé F, Sharp ML, Rasmussen EE, Christy K. The relation between television exposure and executive function among preschoolers. *Dev Psychol* 2014;50(5):1497–506.

10. Crespo CJ, Smit E, Troiano RP, Bartlett SJ, Macera CA, Andersen RE. Television watching, energy intake, and obesity in US children: Results from the third National Health and Nutrition Examination Survey, 1988–1994. *Arch Pediatr Adolesc Med* 2001;155(3):360–65.

11. Zimmerman FJ, Christakis DA. Children's television viewing and cognitive outcomes: A longitudinal analysis of national data. *Arch Pediatr Adolesc Med* 2005;159(7):619–25.

12. Gentzkow M, Shapiro JM. Preschool television viewing and adolescent test scores: Historical evidence from the Coleman Study. *Quart J Econ* 2008;123(1):279–323.

13. Handheld screen time linked with speech delays in young children. Abstract presented at American Academy of Pediatrics, PAS meeting, 2017.

CHAPTER 15: SLOW TALKING, FAST TALKING: LANGUAGE DEVELOPMENT

1. Nelson K. *Narratives from the Crib*. Cambridge, MA: Harvard University Press, 2006.

2. "The MacArthur-Bates Communicative Development Inventory: Words and sentences." https://www.region10.org/r10website/assets/File/Mac%20WS_English.pdf.

3. Available at http://wordbank.stanford.edu/analyses?name=vocab_norms.

4. Rescorla L, Bascome A, Lampard J, Feeny N. Conversational patterns and later talkers at age three. *Appl Psycholinguist* 2001;22:235–51.

5. Rescorla L. Age 17 language and reading outcomes in late-talking toddlers: Support for a dimensional perspective on language delay. *J Speech Lang Hear Res* 2009;52(1):16–30. Rescorla L. Language and reading outcomes to age 9 in late-talking toddlers. *J Speech Lang Hear Res* 2002;45(2):360–71. Rescorla L, Roberts J, Dahlsgaard K. Late talkers at 2: Outcome at age 3. *J Speech Lang Hear Res* 1997;40(3):556–66.

6. Hammer CS, Morgan P, Farkas G, Hillemeier M, Bitetti D, Maczuga S. Late talkers: A population-based study of risk factors and school readiness consequences. *J Speech Lang Hear Res* 2017;60(3): 607–26.

7. Lee J. Size matters: Early vocabulary as a predictor of language and literacy competence. *Appl Psycholinguist* 2011;32(1):69–92.

8. This graph was created by generating some example data based on the mean and standard deviations provided in the paper.

9. Thal DJ et al. Continuity of language abilities: An exploratory study of late and early talking toddlers. *Developmental Neuropsychol* 1997;13(3):239–73.

10. Crain-Thoreson C, Dale PS. Do early talkers become early readers? Linguistic precocity, preschool language, and emergent literacy. *Dev Psychol* 1992;28(3):421.

CHAPTER 16: POTTY TRAINING: STICKERS VS. M&M'S

1. I exclude births after 2013 since those who are born after 2013 and already potty trained by 2017 are a selected group. This exclusion gives time for (most) people to be potty trained.

2. Blum NJ, Taubman B, Nemeth N. Why is toilet training occurring at older ages? A study of factors associated with later training. *J Pediatr* 2004;145(1):107–11.

3. Blum NJ et al. Why is toilet training occurring at older ages?

4. Gilson D, Butler K. A Brief History of the Disposable Diaper. *Mother Jones.* May/June 2008. https://www.motherjones.com/environment/2008/04/brief-history-disposable-diaper.

5. Blum NJ, Taubman B, Nemeth N. Relationship between age at initiation of toilet training and duration of training: A prospective study. *Pediatrics* 2003;111(4):810–14.
6. Vermandel A, Van Kampen M, Van Gorp C, Wyndaele JJ. How to toilet train healthy children? A review of the literature. *Neurourol Urodyn* 2008;27(3):162–66.
7. Vermandel A et al. How to toilet train healthy children?
8. Greer BD, Neidert PL, Dozier CL. A component analysis of toilet-training procedures recommended for young children. *J Appl Behav Anal* 2016;49(1):69–84.
9. Russell K. Among healthy children, what toilet-training strategy is most effective and prevents fewer adverse events (stool withholding and dysfunctional voiding)?: Part A: Evidence-based answer and summary. *Paediatr Child Health* 2008;13(3):201–2.
10. Flensborg-Madsen T, Mortensen EL. Associations of early developmental milestones with adult intelligence. *Child Dev* 2018;89(2):638–48.
11. Taubman B. Toilet training and toileting refusal for stool only: A prospective study. *Pediatrics* 1997;99(1):54–58.
12. Brooks RC, Copen RM, Cox DJ, Morris J, Borowitz S, Sutphen J. Review of the treatment literature for encopresis, functional constipation, and stool-toileting refusal. *Ann Behav Med* 2000;22(3): 260–67.
13. Taubman B, Blum NJ, Nemeth N. Stool toileting refusal: A prospective intervention targeting parental behavior. *Arch Pediatr Adolesc Med* 2003;157(12):1193–96.
14. Taubman B. Toilet training and toileting refusal for stool only.
15. Kliegman R, Nelson WE. *Nelson Textbook of Pediatrics.* Philadelphia: W. B. Saunders Company, 2007.
16. Rugolotto S, Sun M, Boucke L, Calò DG, Tatò L. Toilet training started during the first year of life: A report on elimination signals, stool toileting refusal and completion age. *Minerva Pediatr* 2008;60(1):27–35.

CHAPTER 17: TODDLER DISCIPLINE

1. Bradley SJ, Jadaa DA, Brody J, et al. Brief psychoeducational parenting program: An evaluation and 1-year follow-up. *J Am Acad Child Adolesc Psychiatry* 2003;42(10):1171–78.
2. Porzig-Drummond R, Stevenson RJ, Stevenson C. The 1-2-3 Magic parenting program and its effect on child problem behaviors and dysfunctional parenting: A randomized controlled trial. *Behav Res Ther* 2014;58:52–64.
3. McGilloway S, Bywater T, Ni Mhaille G, Furlong M, Leckey Y, Kelly P, et al. Proving the power of positive parenting: A randomised controlled trial to investigate the effectiveness of the Incredible Years BASIC Parent Training Programme in an Irish context (short-term outcomes). Archways Department of Psychology, NUI Maynooth. 2009.
4. Haroon M. Commentary on "Behavioural and cognitive-behavioural group-based parenting programmes for early-onset conduct problems in children aged 3 to 12 years." *Evid Based Child Health* 2013;8(2):693–94.
5. MacKenzie MJ, Nicklas E, Brooks-Gunn J, Waldfogel J. Who spanks infants and toddlers? Evidence from the fragile families and child well-being study. *Child Youth Serv Rev* 2011;33(8):1364–73.
6. Maguire-Jack K, Gromoske AN, Berger LM. Spanking and child development during the first 5 years of life. *Child Dev* 2012;83(6):1960–77.
7. Gershoff ET, Sattler KMP, Ansari A. Strengthening causal estimates for links between spanking and children's externalizing behavior problems. *Psychol Sci* 2018;29(1):110–20.
8. Ferguson CJ. Spanking, corporal punishment and negative long-term outcomes: A meta-analytic review of longitudinal studies. *Clin Psychol Rev* 2013;33(1):196–208. Gershoff ET, Grogan-Kaylor A. Spanking and child outcomes: Old controversies and new meta-analyses. *J Fam Psychol* 2016;30(4): 453–69.
9. Afifi TO, Ford D, Gershoff ET, et al. Spanking and adult mental health impairment: The case for the designation of spanking as an adverse childhood experience. *Child Abuse Negl* 2017;71:24–31.

CHAPTER 18: EDUCATION

1. For a review of this literature, see Price J, Kalil A. The effect of parental time investments on children's cognitive achievement: Evidence from natural within-family variation. *Child Dev*, forthcoming.

2. Bus AG, Van IJzendoorn MH, Pelligrini AD. Joint book reading makes for success in learning to read: A meta-analysis on intergenerational transmission of literacy. *Rev Educ Res* 1995;65(1):1–21. Sloat EA, Letourneau NL, Joschko JR, Schryer EA, Colpitts JE. Parent-mediated reading interventions with children up to four years old: A systematic review. *Issues Compr Pediatr Nurs* 2015;38(1):39–56.

3. Mendelsohn AL, Cates CB, Weisleder A, Johnson SB, Seery AM, Canfield CF, et al. Reading aloud, play, and social-emotional development. *Pediatrics* 2018;e20173393.

4. Price J, Kalil A. The effect of parental time investments on children's cognitive achievement.

5. Hutton JS, Horowitz-Kraus T, Mendelsohn AL, Dewitt T, Holland SK. Home reading environment and brain activation in preschool children listening to stories. *Pediatrics* 2015;136(3):466–78.

6. Whitehurst GJ, Falco FL, Lonigan CJ, Fischel JE, DeBaryshe BD, Valdez-Menchaca MC, Caulfield M. Accelerating language development through picture book reading. *Dev Psych* 1988;24(4):552–59.

7. Available at http://www.intellbaby.com/teach-your-baby-to-read.

8. Neuman SB, Kaefer T, Pinkham A, Strouse G. Can babies learn to read? A randomized trial of baby media. *J Educ Psych* 2014;106(3):815–30.

9. Wolf GM. Letter-sound reading: Teaching preschool children print-to-sound processing. *Early Child Educ J* 2016;44(1):11–19.

10. Pennington BF, Johnson C, Welsh MC. Unexpected reading precocity in a normal preschooler: Implications for hyperlexia. *Brain Lang* 1987;30(1):165–80. Fletcher-Flinn CM, Thompson GB. Learning to read with underdeveloped phonemic awareness but lexicalized phonological recoding: A case study of a 3-year-old. *Cognition* 2000;74(2):177–208.

11. Welsh MC, Pennington BF, Rogers S. Word recognition and comprehension skills in hyperlexic children. *Brain Lang* 1987;32(1):76–96.

12. Lillard AS. Preschool children's development in classic Montessori, supplemented Montessori, and conventional programs. *J Sch Psychol* 2012;50(3):379–401. Miller LB, Bizzell RP. Long-term effects of four preschool programs: Sixth, seventh, and eighth grades. *Child Dev* 1983;54(3):727–41.

13. Suggate SP, Schaughency EA, Reese E. Children learning to read later catch up to children reading earlier. *Early Child Res Q* 2013;28(1):33–48. Elben J, Nicholson T. Does learning the alphabet in kindergarten give children a head start in the first year of school? A comparison of children's reading progress in two first grade classes in state and Montessori schools in Switzerland. *Aust J Learn Diffic* 2017;22(2):95–108.

CHAPTER 19: INTERNAL POLITICS

1. Dunn J. You will hate your husband after your kid is born. Available at http://www.slate.com/articles/life/family/2017/05/happy_mother_s_day_you_will_hate_your_husband_after_having_a_baby.html.

2. This chapter will really only scratch the surface of the marital issues that arise. For a more complete and nuanced discussion, see (among others) http://www.brigidschulte.com/books/overwhelmed.

3. Rollins B, Feldman H. Marital satisfaction over the family life cycle. *J Marriage Fam* 1970;32(1):23.

4. Lawrence E, Rothman AD, Cobb RJ, Rothman MT, Bradbury TN. Marital satisfaction across the transition to parenthood. *J Fam Psychol* 2008;22(1):41–50. Twenge JM, Campbell WK, Foster CA. Parenthood and marital satisfaction: A meta-analytic review. *J Marriage Fam* 2003;65:574–83.

5. Lawrence E et al. Marital satisfaction across the transition to parenthood.

6. Available at https://www.bls.gov/news.release/atus2.t01.htm.

7. Archer E, Shook RP, Thomas DM, et al. 45-year trends in women's use of time and household management energy expenditure. *PLoS ONE* 2013;8(2):e56620.

8. Schneider D. Market earnings and household work: New tests of gender performance theory. *J Marriage Fam* 2011;73(4):845–60.

9. Dribe M, Stanfors M. Does parenthood strengthen a traditional household division of labor? Evidence from Sweden. *J Marriage Fam* 2009;71:33–45.

10. Chan RW, Brooks RC, Raboy B, Patterson CJ. Division of labor among lesbian and heterosexual parents: Associations with children's adjustment. *J Fam Psychol* 1998;12(3):402–19. Goldberg AE, Smith JZ, Perry-Jenkins M. The division of labor in lesbian, gay, and heterosexual new adoptive parents. *J Marriage Fam* 2012;74:812–28.

11. Wheatley D, Wu Z. Dual careers, time-use and satisfaction levels: Evidence from the British Household Panel Survey. *Indus Rel J* 2014;45:443–64.

12. Available at http://www.brigidschulte.com/books/overwhelmed.

13. Schneidewind-Skibbe A, Hayes RD, Koochaki PE, Meyer J, Dennerstein L. The frequency of sexual intercourse reported by women: A review of community-based studies and factors limiting their conclusions. *J Sex Med* 2008;5(2):301–35. McDonald E, Woolhouse H, Brown SJ. Consultation about sexual health issues in the year after childbirth: A cohort study. *Birth* 2015;42(4):354–61.

14. Johnson MD, Galambos NL, Anderson JR. Skip the dishes? Not so fast! Sex and housework revisited. *J Fam Psychol* 2016;30(2):203–13.

15. Medina AM, Lederhos CL, Lillis TA. Sleep disruption and decline in marital satisfaction across the transition to parenthood. *Fam Syst Health* 2009;27(2):153–60.

16. Cordova JV, Fleming CJ, Morrill MI, et al. The Marriage Checkup: A randomized controlled trial of annual relationship health checkups. *J Consult Clin Psychol* 2014;82(4):592–604.

17. Cordova JV et al. The Marriage Checkup. Schulz MS, Cowan CP, Cowan PA. Promoting healthy beginnings: A randomized controlled trial of a preventive intervention to preserve marital quality during the transition to parenthood. *J Consult Clin Psychol* 2006;74(1):20–31. Cowan CP, Cowan PA, Barry J. Couples' groups for parents of preschoolers: Ten-year outcomes of a randomized trial. *J Fam Psychol* 2011;25(2):240–50.

CHAPTER 20: EXPANSIONS

1. The other common approach here is to use child gender. If a family has two children of the same gender first, they are more likely to try for a third. It is therefore possible to compare families with, say, a boy and a girl first to those with two boys, and the one with two boys is more likely to have a third kid, giving you some random variation in family size.

2. Black SE, Devereux PJ, Salvanes KG. The more the merrier? The effect of family size and birth order on children's education. *Q J Econ* 2005;120(2):669–700; Black SE, Devereux PJ, Salvanes KG. Small family, smart family? Family size and the IQ scores of young men. *J Hum Resourc* 2010;45(1):33–58.

3. In the second of these papers, the authors find that when the higher family size is a result of having twins, IQ scores do suffer, but not if the higher family size is a result of gender of the first children, suggesting that it is the surprise that matters, not the size.

4. Polit DF, Falbo T. Only children and personality development: A quantitative review. *J Marriage Fam* 1987;309–25.

5. Coo H, Brownell MD, Ruth C, Flavin M, Au W, Day AG. Interpregnancy interval and adverse perinatal outcomes: A record-linkage study using the Manitoba Population Research Data Repository. *J Obstet Gynaecol Can* 2017;39(6):420–33.

6. Shachar BZ, Mayo JA, Lyell DJ, et al. Interpregnancy interval after live birth or pregnancy termination and estimated risk of preterm birth: A retrospective cohort study. *BJOG* 2016;123(12):2009–17. Koullali B, Kamphuis EI, Hof MH, et al. The effect of interpregnancy interval on the recurrence rate of spontaneous preterm birth: A retrospective cohort study. *Am J Perinatol* 2017;34(2):174–82.

7. Class QA, Rickert ME, Oberg AS, et al. Within-family analysis of interpregnancy interval and adverse birth outcomes. *Obstet Gynecol* 2017;130(6):1304–11.

8. Buckles KS, Munnich EL. Birth spacing and sibling outcomes. *J Human Res* 2012;47:613–42.

9. Conde-Agudelo A, Rosas-Bermudez A, Norton MH. Birth spacing and risk of autism and other neurodevelopmental disabilities: A systematic review. *Pediatrics* 2016;137(5).

INDEX

abdominal massages, 43
abdominal pain, after childbirth, 48
acetaminophen (Tylenol), 38, 39, 105, 143, 144
Adverse Effects of Vaccines: Evidence and Causality, 139–44
African American boys, and vaccinations, 304*n*
alcohol consumption
  breastfeeding and, 104–5
  SIDS and, 119, *119,* 126
allergies (allergic reactions). *See also* food allergies
  breastfeeding and, 35, *67,* 79, *86*
  early exposure, 188–91, 199–200, 203
  germ exposure and, 37
  low-allergen diet, and breastfeeding, 35, 103
  to vaccinations, 142, 144, 147
American Academy of Pediatrics (AAP)
  circumcision guidelines, 11
  sleep guidelines, 111–12, 123, 124, 131
  starting solid foods, 191–92
  TV (screen) time guidelines, 218
  vaccination guidelines, 138–39
American College of Obstetricians and Gynecologists, 49
anemia, 203
antibiotics
  colds and, 215–16
  in the eye, 26–27
  for mastitis, 96
antidepressants, 56, 105–6
artificial nipples, 96–98
Asana, 184
Asian-heritage infants, and jaundice, 25
attachment parenting (AP), 167, 173–75, 178, 179

autism
  birth spacing and, 287
  early reading and, 264
  vaccines and, 136–37, 139–40, 147

"baby blues," 52–57
Baby Einstein, 218, 219–20
"baby-friendly hospitals," 13–14
baby-led weaning, 193–94, 203
baby monitors, 121, 126–27
baby "sighs," 31
Baby Wordsworth, 220
back sleep position, 112, 114–17
"Back to Sleep" campaign, 112, 116–17
baths (bathing) of newborns, 7–9
"Bayesian statistics," 225–26, 227
Becker, Gary, 283
bed sharing. *See* co-sleeping
bedtime routine, 176
bedtime schedules, 128–29, 133–34
beer, 101, 104–5
behavioral problems, 211
  childcare and, 161–65, 166–67, 170
  discipline and. *See* toddler discipline
best parenting advice, 290–91
bilirubin, 22, 23–24
binge drinking, 104–5
birth. *See* childbirth
birth control, 50–51
birth order, 284
birth spacing, 285–87
birth weight, 18, 115, 126, 286. *See also* infant weight loss
bleeding
  after childbirth, 43, 44, 58
  vitamin K shot and, 26
blood tests, 12

blue light therapy, 23–24, 25
body temperature, and newborn baths, 8
brain development. *See* cognitive
    development; IQ
brain injuries, 22, 31
  vaccinations and, 137, 138
breastfeeding, xx–xxii, 61–62, 65–110
  benefits for mother, 83–85
  bottom line summaries, 87, 109–10
  "claimed" benefits of, 66–68, *67*, 83–85
  colic and crying, 35
  contraception use and, 50–51
  co-sleeping and, 120–21
  diet for, 35, 103–6, 196–97
  early-life health and, 74–77
  how-to-guide. *See* breastfeeding,
    how-to guide
  infant weight loss and, 18, 20–21
  IQ and, 68–69, 81–83
  later health and, 79–81
  parental education and income, 68–69
  "rooming in," 14, 15–16, 91
  SIDS and, 77–79
  skin-to-skin contact and, 8, 90–91, 109
  solid food introduction and, 191–92
  studies. *See* breastfeeding studies
breastfeeding, how-to guide, 88–110
  bottom line summary, 109–10
  general interventions, 90–91
  hospital versus in-home education, 91
  latching on, *92*, 92–96
  milk supply. *See* milk supply
  nipple confusion, 96–98, 109
  nipple pain, 89, 95–96, 102, 109
  oversupply, 89, 99, 102
  pumping, 89, 106–9
breastfeeding studies, xx–xxii, 68–69, 73–74
  benefits, 74–87
  bottom line summary, 87
  data and research methods, xxi–xxii, 70–73
  the verdict, 85–87
breast pumps, 89, 106–9
breast reductions, and milk supply, 101–2
Bringing Up Bébé (Druckerman), 252
bris ceremony, 9
British Medical Journal, 115, 118, 121–22
broccoli, 103, 195, 198
bumpers, 112, 124–25, 127

caesarean section (C-section), 5
  average weight, *19*, 19–20
  peeing, 45–46

  physical recovery from, 42, 43, 46–47, 48,
    49, 58
caffeine, 106
California
  newborn blood screening, 12
  parental leave provisions, 154
cancer, 11
  breastfeeding and, 80, 85, 300–301*n*
carrots, 192, 196
case-control studies, 72–73, 74, 78, 115, 118
cauliflower, 103, 251
causality, xxi, 15, 62–63, 82, 139–40, 151–52, 196
Centers for Disease Control, 138–39
cerebral palsy (CP), 211, 216
chest pains, after childbirth, 48
chicken pox, 146
chicken pox vaccine, 135, 143, 146
childbirth, 3–4, 5. *See also* caesarean section;
    vaginal birth
  bleeding after, 44–45
  delivery room, 25–27
  emotional health after, 52–58
  lingering consequences after, 46–48
  peeing and pooping after, 45–46
  physical recovery from. *See* physical recovery
    from childbirth
  serious complications after, 48
childbirth classes, 41
childcare, 159–70
  bottom line summary, 170
  day-care option, 160, 161–65
  day care vs. nanny, 166–70
  decision tree, *160*, 160–61
  nanny option, 160, 165–66
  work considerations, 155–57, 168
Child Development, 257, 261
child-led potty training, 244–46
choking, 194, 200
chore allocation, 276–78
Christakis, Dimitri, 222–23
circumcision, 6–7, 9–12, 27
  benefits, 10–11
  cultural traditions of, 9–10
  pain relief and, 11–12
  risks, 9–10
  U.S. rates of, 9
Clostridium botulinum, 201
coffee (caffeine), 106
cognitive behavioral therapy, 56
cognitive development, 211. *See also* IQ
  breastfeeding and, *67*, 68–69, *86*, 87
  childcare and, 161–65, 166–67, 170

reading to children and, 262
sleep and, 117, 123
TV exposure and, 218
cognitive dissonance, xxiii
colds, 214–16
breastfeeding and, 76, 77
colic, 32–35, 39
as self-limiting, 34, 39
statistics on, 33
treatments, 34–35
colostrum, 18, 99
comparative advantage, 276–77
complications, after childbirth, 5, 48
"confidence intervals," 76
"constrained optimization," xxiii
contraception, 50–51
cooking
meal kits, xviii–xix
meal prep, xviii–xix
two-dinner option, xviii, xix
cord clamping, delayed, 25–26, 27
cortisol, 180
co-sleeping, xvii, 112, 114, 117–21, 126–27
benefits, 120–21
risks, death rates, 118–20, *119*
sleep training and, 173–74
counseling programs, 279
couple therapy, 279
cow's milk, 199, 200
crankiness, and vaccinations, 143–44
crib bumpers, 112, 124–25, 127
cribs, 111–12, 117–18, 124
no-stuff-in-the-crib recommendation, 112,
124–25, 127
crying
colic and, 32–35
swaddled babies and, 301
"cry it out" method, 173–76
benefits, 177, 187
bottom line summary, 187
harm, 177–81
methods, 175–76, 182–83

data collection, 35–37, 40
sleep apps, 131–32
day care, 160, 161–65, 264–65
bottom line summary, 170
decision tree, *160*, 160–61
evaluating quality, 161–65, 265
nannies vs., 166–70
daytime sleep, 129–33, 134, 183
decision-theory, 160–61

deformational plagiocephaly, 117
dehydration, 18, 21, 35–36, 45
delayed cord clamping, 25–26, 27
delayed milk onset, 99–101, *100*
delayed motor development, 210–12, 216
delayed talking, 234–37
delivery room, 25–27. *See also* childbirth
physical recovery from childbirth, 42–43
"demographic transition," 283
depression. *See* postpartum depression
developmental psychology, 219
diapers, 238, 241, 243–44, 247–48
diarrhea, 75, 79, 81, 216
diet. *See also* solid food introduction
for breastfeeding, 35, 103–6, 196–97
discipline. *See* toddler discipline
Dr. Spock's Baby and Child Care, 86–87, 98, 115
domperidone, 101
dorsal penile nerve block (DPNB), 12
doulas, 55, 91, 93
Down syndrome, 212
drugs, and breastfeeding, 105–6
dryness
nighttime, 247–48
vaginal, 51
DTaP vaccines, 137, 141, 142

ear infections, 76–77, 79, *86*, 215
Early Childhood Longitudinal Study, 236
early exposure to allergens, 188–91,
199–200, 203
early-life health, and breastfeeding, 74–77
early reading, 263
economic approach to decision-making, xvii–xx
eczema, 75, 77
Edinburgh Postnatal Depression Scale, 53,
54, 55
education, 259–68
bottom line summary, 268
learning to read, 263–64
reading to your child, 261–62
types of preschool, 264–68
"Elimination Communication" potty training,
244, 248–49
elimination diet, 35
emotional health after childbirth, 52–58. *See
also* postpartum depression
"encouragement design," 70–71, 74–76
"endpoint-oriented" potty training, 243–44
epidurals, 43, 45, 100
evidence-based parenting, 76, 208, 245,
251, 252

exchange transfusion, 25
exercise, after childbirth, 48–49, 58
expansions, 282–88
    birth spacing, 285–87
    bottom line summary, 288
    number of children, 283–84
Expecting Better (Oster), xix, xxiv, 25, 223
"Extinction" method, 175–76, 182
Extinction with Parental Presence, 176, 182
eye antibiotics, 26–27

Facebook, xvii, 6, 154, 239, 271
fainting, after vaccinations, 142
family expansions. *See* expansions
Family Medical Leave Act (FMLA), 154, 155
febrile seizures, 143, 146–47
fenugreek, 90, 101
Ferber, Richard, *Solve Your Child's Sleep Problems*, 129–30, 172, 173, 182
fertility problems, 285, 287
fertility rates, 283
fevers
    germ exposure and, 38–39
    vaccinations and, 143, 146–47
fingernail cutting, 140
first postbirth bowel movement, 45–46
first three days, 5–27
    bottom line summary, 27
    delivery room, 25–27
    the expected, 7–17
    the unexpected, 17–25
first weeks at home, 28–40
    bottom line summary, 39–40
    colic and crying, 32–35
    data collection, 35–37
    germ exposure, 37–39
    swaddling, 29–32
first year, 61–203
    breastfeeding, 65–110
    childcare, 159–70
    sleep, 111–34, 171–87
    solid food introduction, 188–203
    vaccinations, 135–47
    work decision, 148–58
fish, high-mercury, and breastfeeding, 103
flat head, 117
flavor exposure, 195–96
food. *See* diet; solid food introduction
food allergies, 192, 199–200. *See also* peanut allergies
    early exposure, 188–91, 199–200, 203
food neophobia, 197–98

food refusal, 197–98
"forbidden foods" list, 200–201
formula, 68
    colic and crying, 34–35, 103
Freemie, 106–7
free-rider problem, 146
"frequentist statistics," 225
friendships, and breastfeeding, 67, 83–84
fruits, 191, 194, 195, 196, 200
fruit juice, 200
fruit purees, 200
fundal massage, 43

gender differences
    household work, 276–77
    language development, 229–30, 233–34, 237
    work and parenting, 149, 150
general equilibrium theory, 33
Gentzkow, Matthew, 223–24
germ exposure, 37–39, 40
Graduated Extinction, 176, 182, 184
grapes, 200
group couples therapy, 279
gua sha therapy, 102

head control, 210, 211, 214
Head Start, 167, 265, 268
health economics, xvii
"healthy diet," 195–96
Healthy Sleep Habits, Happy Child (Weissbluth), 129–30, 172–73, 182–83, 184, 185
hearing loss, 13
hearing tests, 13
heel pricks, 6, 12, 23
hemorrhoids, 47
hepatitis B vaccines, 135, 147
herbal remedies, for milk supply, 101–2
"herd immunity," 145–46
hip dysplasia, 31
HIV, 11
home front, 271–91
    family expansions, 282–88
    marital-happiness problems, 273–81
honey, 200–201
Hooker, Brian, 304*n*
hospital
    blood and hearing tests, 12–13
    delivery room, 25–27
    newborn baths, 7–9
    "rooming in," 13–17
hospital blankets, 29–30

hospital nurseries, 13–14, 16, 17
household-work time, 276–78
HPV vaccine, 135
hydration, 106
hygiene hypothesis, 37–38
hyperlexia, 264

ibuprofen, 105
IKEA, 159, 178
illness, 214–16
incontinence, 47
Incredible Years, 252, 255
"infant attachment," 167
infant botulism, 200–201
infant crankiness, and vaccinations, 143–44
infant health, and birth spacing, 285–87
infantile colic, 32–35
infant weight loss, 17–21, 27
    average, *19*, 19–21
    supplementation for, 20–21
Institute of Medicine (IOM), 139–44
insufficient glandular tissue (IGT), 101–2
IQ (intelligence quotient)
    birth order and, 284
    birth spacing and, 285
    breastfeeding and, 68–69, 81–83
    language development and, 235–36
    potty training and, 246
    TV watching and, 222
iron, 202, 203
Israel, and peanut allergies, 188–89

jaundice, 21–25, 27
    primary sign of, 23–24
    treatment options, 23–25
Journal of Child and Adolescent Psychiatry,
    254–55
Journal of Pediatrics, 125, 240
Journal of Sleep Research, 132
*Journal of the American Medical
    Association,* 116
Judaism, and circumcision and, 12
juice, 200
juvenile arthritis, 80
juvenile diabetes, 80, 300*n*

kernicterus, 22–23
kitchen sponge etiquette, 273

Lack, Gideon, 188–90, 191
lactation, 98–102
lactation consultants, 5, 18, 91, 95–96

Lancet, 137–38, 144, 304*n*
language development, 228–37
    Baby Einstein products, 219–20
    bottom line summary, 237
    childcare and, 161–65, 166–67, 170
    distribution of words, 230–34
    first words, 229
    gender differences, 229–30, 233–34, 237
    timing of, 234–37
    vocabulary size, 231–34
lanolin cream, 95
latch, the (latching on), 66, 88, *92*, 92–96
    common interventions, 93–95
later health, and breastfeeding, 79–81
leukemia, 300–301*n*
Li, Dawn, 23, 184, 209, 214, 290–91
lingering consequences, after childbirth, 46–48
Lion Gets Potty Trained, The, 245–46
lip ties, 94–95
longitudinal studies, 161
loose skin, 46
low-allergen diet, and breastfeeding, 35, 103
lumbar puncture, 38, 40

MacArthur-Bates Communicative
    Development Inventories (MB-CDI),
    231–34
"marginal value," 150, 157, 168
marital-happiness problems, 273–81
    bottom line summary, 281
    household-work time, 276–78
    sex-chore relationship, 276, 277–78
    solutions, 278–80
"marriage checkup," 279
mastitis, 96, 102
maternal hemorrhage, 44
maternity leave, 152, 153–55, 158
meal kits, xviii–xix
measles, 135, 136, 138, 142
measles inclusion body encephalitis, 142
measles vaccine, 135
meatal stenosis, 10
medications, and breastfeeding, 105–6
menstrual pads, 41
mesh underwear, 41–42
"meta-analyses," 118
milk supply, 89, 98–102, 110
    days until milk production, 99–100, *100*
    drinking and, 105
    feedback loop and, 99–100, 110
    herbal remedies for, 101–2
    how to increase, 101–2

milk supply *(cont.)*
 oversupply, 89, 99, 102
 undersupply, 89, 99–102, *100*, 107
Miracle Blanket, xiii, 30
mitten injuries, 28–29
MMR vaccine, 137–38, 139–47, 304*n*
Mommy Wars, xxii–xxiii, 61
 vaccinations, 135–36
 work decision, 148
Montessori education, 266–67
"more chores, less sex," 276, 277–78
"more chores, more sex," 276, 277–78
Mother's Encyclopedia in Six Volumes, 98
motor delays, 210–12, 216
multiple sclerosis, 141
multivitamins, 202
"mummy tummy," 46
muscular dystrophy, 212

nannies, 160, 165–66
 bottom line summary, 170
 day care vs., 166–70
 decision tree, *160*, 160–61
 hiring, 165–66
 sharing, 168–69
naps (napping), 183
 age range, 130, 134
 amount of, 129–33, *131*
Narratives from the Crib (Nelson), 228–29
Narvaez, Darcia, 174
Nathanson, Laura, 215
National Childhood Vaccine Injury Act of
 1986, 137
necrotizing enterocolitis (NEC), 75
Nelson, Katherine, 228–29
neonatal abstinence syndrome, 14–15, 31
nettle tea, 89, 101
neurological diseases, 212
newborn baths, 7–9
newborns
 first three days. *See* first three days
 first weeks. *See* first weeks at home
New England Journal of Medicine, 189–90
New Jersey, parental leave provisions, 154
New York, parental leave provisions, 154
NICHD Study of Early Child Care and Youth
 Development, 161–65, 166–67
nighttime dryness, 247–48
nighttime sleep, 129–33, 134
nipple confusion, 96–98, 109
nipple pain, 89, 95–96, 102, 109
nipple shields, 93–94

nipple yeast infections, 95
No-Cry Sleep Solution, The (Pantley), 172, 173
nuts, 200

obesity, and breastfeeding, 79–80
observational studies, 71–72, 73–74
1-2-3 Magic, 252, 254–55
only child, 284
open-ended questions, 262, 263
opioids, and breastfeeding, 105–6
"opportunity costs," xviii–xix, 226
optimal choices, xxiii
orphanage literature, 174–75, 179
overheating, xiv–xv, 31–32, 115
oversupply, 89, 99, 102

pacifiers, 14, 96–98, *97*
painful nipples, 89, 95–96, 102, 109
painkillers, and breastfeeding, 105–6
pain relief, and circumcision, 11–12
pains, after childbirth, 48
Paltrow, Gwyneth, 102
Pantley, Elizabeth, *The No-Cry Sleep Solution,*
 172, 173
parental discipline, 252–53. *See also* toddler
 discipline
parental education and income
 breastfeeding and, 68–69
 language development and, 235
parental leave, 152, 153–55, 158
parental work, 148–58
 bottom line summary, 158
 budgeting issues, 155–57
 impacts of parental employment on child
 outcomes, 151–53
 making a choice, 157–58
 structuring the decision, 149–51
parenthood, 271–72
 expansions, 282–88
 marital-happiness problems, 273–81
parenting decisions, xxiii–xxiv, 4, 61–62
 economic approach to decision-making,
 xvii–xx
 use of data, xx–xxiv
parenting decision tree, *160*, 160–61
Parton, Dolly, 260
peanut allergies, 188–91, *190*, 199
peanut timing, 188–91, 199–200
Pediatrics, 18
peeing, after childbirth, 45–46, 48
penile cancer, 11
penis sensitivity, and circumcision, 10

pertussis, 145–46
pertussis vaccine, 137, 145–46
phenylalanine, 12
phenylketonuria (PKU), 12
phimosis, 11
phonics, 264
phototherapy, 23–24, 25
physical milestones, 209–16
  bottom line summary, 216
  developmental milestones, *212*, 212–14, *213*
  distributions, 210–11
  early intervention, 209–10
  illness, 214–16
  motor delays, 210–12, 216
physical recovery from childbirth, 41–51
  bottom line summary, 42
  in the delivery room, 42–43
  exercise and sex, 48–51
  in the recovery room and beyond, 44–48
picky/fussy eaters, 197–98, 202
pooping, after childbirth, 45–46
Portable Pediatrician for Parents, The
  (Nathanson), 215
"positive parenting," 261
postpartum anxiety, 52, 56
postpartum depression, 52–57, 58
  breastfeeding and, 84–85, 105–6
  diagnosis, 53, *54*, 55
  exercise for, 49
  risk factors, 53
  treatment, 55–56
postpartum psychosis, 52, 56
postpartum shortness of breath, 48
potty training, 208, 238–49
  appropriate age to start, 238–43, *240*,
    242, 249
  bottom line summary, 249
  completion of, 242, *242*, 249
  duration of, *242*, 242–43
  "Elimination Communication" potty
    training, 244, 248–49
  methods, 243–46, 258
  problems and extensions, 246–48
premature birth
  breastfeeding and, 93–94
  delayed cord cutting, 26, 27
  maternity leave and, 154
  SIDS and, 78, 113, 117, 126
preschool, 259–60
  types of, 264–68
preterm birth, 287, 288
"prior beliefs," 141, 225

probiotics, 34, 39
PROBIT (Promotion of Breastfeeding
    Intervention Trial), 74–76, 79–80, 82–83
prodigious early reading, 263
prone sleeping position, 302–3*n*
pumping, 89, 106–9
pumping bras, 108
pumping wipes, 108
punishment. *See* toddler discipline

"quantity-quality" trade-off, 283

randomized controlled trials, 70–73, 189
  breastfeeding, 35, 63, 74–76, 79–80
  delayed cord cutting, 26
  "rooming in," 15–16
rashes, 75
reading, 259–60
  bottom line summary, 268
  learning to read, 263–64
  in preschool, 267–68
  to your child, 261–62
Reggio Emilia-inspired schools, 266
religious male circumcision, 6–7, 12
Rescorla, Leslie, 235–36
research methods, 70–73
Rhode Island
  parental leave, 154
  reading program, 260
rice cereal, 191, 192, 196, 203
rickets, 201–2
Rock 'n Play Sleeper, xiii, xx
rolling ability, 210, 212–13
Romanian orphanages, 174–75, 179
"rooming in," 13–17, 27
  benefits, 14–15
  risks, 15, 16
room sharing, 112, 121–23, 126–27

same-sex couples, 277
schedules. *See also* sleep schedules
  data collection, 35–37, 40
  vaccinations, 146–47
school readiness, and Head Start, 167, 265, 268
screen time. *See* TV time
Sears, William, 173–74
Sesame Street, 217–18, 220–21, 226
sex
  after childbirth, 50–51, 58
  chore allocation and, 276, 277–78
sex stereotypes, 149, 153
sexually transmitted infections (STIs), 11, 25, 26

Shapiro, Finn, xiv–xv, 289
  breastfeeding, 66, 79–80, 83, 107
  discipline issues, 251
  first few days, 8–9, 14, 21–22, 25, 43, 47, 50
  language development, 229, 230–31
  potty training, 245
  preschool, 259–60
  sleep considerations, 111, 112, 126–27,
    128–29, 133, 173, 184–86
  solid food introduction, 192, 193, 198, 201
  TV viewing, 220, 221
Shapiro, Jesse, xiv, xviii, 159, 289
  childbirth classes, 41
  data collection, 36
  first days of Finn's life, 14
  first days of Penelope's life, 3, 6
  internal politics, 273, 274, 279–80
  potty training, 238
  sleep considerations, 112, 128–29
  TV access and test scores, 223–24
  vaccinations, 143
Shapiro, Penelope, xvi, xviii, xix–xx, 274, 289
  breastfeeding, 65–66, 88, 107
  discipline, 250–51
  first few days, xii, 3–4, 14, 17–18, 20, 23
  first weeks at home, 28, 32–33, 35–36, 52
  France vacation, 290–91
  language development, 229
  physical milestones, 209–10
  sleep considerations, 111, 112, 126–27,
    128–29, 133, 184–86
  solid food introduction, 190, 191, 195, 201
  vaccinations and crankiness, 143
shortness of breath, after childbirth, 48
sibling expansions. *See* expansions
sibling studies, 71–72, 73–74, 80, 82, 144
side sleeping, 116–17
SIDS. *See* sudden infant death syndrome
simethicone, 34
Singh, Prerna, 136–37
skin-to-skin contact, 8, 90–91
sleep, 111–34, 171–87
  AAP guidelines, 111–12, 123, 124, 131
  books about, 129–30, 172–73
  bottom line summaries, 127, 134, 187
  duration, 129–33, *131*, 171–72
  location. *See* sleep location
  marital satisfaction and, 279
  position. *See* sleep position
  risks, 113–14
  risks and making choices, 125–27
  schedule. *See* sleep schedules

  swaddled babies and, 30–31
  training. *See* sleep training
sleep location. *See also* cribs
  co-sleeping, 112, 114, 117–21
  room sharing, 112, 121–23
  sharing sofa with adult, 123, 125
Sleep Medicine Reviews, 179
sleep patterns, 131–32
sleep position, 112
  on the back, 112, 114–17
  rolling over, 116–17
  SIDS and, 112, 113–25
  on stomach, 112, 114–16
sleep schedules, 128–34
  age range, 130, 134
  amount of sleep, 129–33, *131*, 171–72
  bottom line summary, 134
  duration of sleep, 129–33, *131*
  wake-up times, 120, 133
sleep training, 171–87
  appropriate age to start, 182–83
  benefits, 177
  bottom line summary, 187
  consistency, 182, 184, 187
  "crying it out," 173–76, 177–81
  efficacy, 175–76
  philosophies, 172–75
  which method and when, 175–76, 182–83
smartphone parenting, 131–32
smoking
  breastfeeding and, 80, 100
  SIDS and, 78, 119, *119*, 125, 126
soda, 200
sofa sleeping deaths, 123, 125
solid food introduction, 188–203
  AAP guidelines, 191–92
  baby-led weaning, 193–94
  bottom line summary, 203
  flavor exposure, 195–96
  "forbidden foods" list, 200–201
  peanut timing, 188–91
  picky/fussy eaters, 197–98, 202
  timing, 191–94
  waiting between foods, 192
  what to eat, 194–98
"solve the tree," 160–61
Solve Your Child's Sleep Problems (Ferber),
  129–30, 172, 173, 182
Somali immigrant community, measles
  outbreak, 136, 138
sore nipples, 89, 95–96, 102, 109
spanking, 256–57, 258

spina bifida, 212

spinal tap, 38, 40

Spock's Baby and Child Care, 86–87, 98, 115

sponge baths, 8, 27

SpongeBob SquarePants, 225–26

Square One Television, 217

SSRIs (selective serotonin reuptake inhibitors), 106

standing, 214

"stay-at-home dads," 149

stomach sleep position, 112, 114–16

stool softeners, 45

stool toileting refusal, 241, 246–47, 249

"stress resistance," and breastfeeding, 83–84

sudden infant death syndrome (SIDS), 119–25

  breastfeeding and, 77–79

  causes of, 113

  co-sleeping and, 112, 114, 117–21

  cribs and, 117–18

  death rates by behavior, 118–20, *119*, 122, 126

  risks and making choices, 125–27

  room sharing and, 112, 121–23

  sleep position and, 112, 113–25

  swaddling and, 31

"surprise" births, 284, 285

swaddle blankets, 30

swaddling, 29–32, 39

  benefits, 30–31

  breaking the habit, xii–xv

  cautions, 31–32

Sweden, 159–60, 276, 286

take-out, xviii, xix

tantrums, 250–51, 253

taste, 195–97

Teach Your Baby to Read, 263

Tennessee, reading program, 260

test scores

  birth spacing and, 287

  early motor delays and, 211

  early reading and, 235, 237

  parental education and, 235

  parental work and, 152–53

  reading to child and, 261

  TV viewing and, 218, 222–24, 226

toddler discipline, 250–58

  bottom line summary, 258

  consistency in, 253–54

  parenting approaches to, 252–56

  rewards and punishments, 252–54

  spanking, 256–57

toddlers, 207–68

  education, 259–68

  language development, 228–37

  physical milestones, 209–16

  potty training, 238–49

  TV time, 217–27

tongue ties, 94–95

Triple P-Positive Parenting Program, 252

TV time, 217–27

  AAP guidelines, 218

  "Bayesian statistics," 225–26

  bottom line summary, 227

  harm question, 221–24

  learning from, 219–21

type 1 diabetes, 80, 300*n*

umbilical cord, delayed cord clamping, 25–26

undersupply, 89, 99–101, *100*, 107

  how to increase, 101–2

unplanned births, 284, 285

urinary tract infections (UTIs), 10, 38, 80

uterine ("fundal") massage, 43

vaccinations, 135–47

  background, 136–39

  bottom line summary, 147

  delayed schedules, 146–47

  efficacy, 145–46

  rates, 135, 136, 145–46

  safety, 139–44

  scientific consensus on, 136

vaginal birth, 5

  average weight, *19*, 19–20

  peeing, 45–46

  physical recovery from, 42–43, 45–46, 48, 49, 58

vaginal discharge, after childbirth, 48

vaginal dryness, 51

vaginal tearing, 42–43, 49, 50, 58

vegetables, 191, 195–97

vernix, 7

vitamin C deficiency, 202

vitamin D supplements, 201–3

vitamin K shots, 26

vitamin supplementation, 201–3

vocabulary development, 219–20

vocabulary size, 231–34, *232, 233, 234,* 237

Wakefield, Andrew, 137–38, 144, 304*n*

wake-up times, 120, 133, 134

Waldorf schools, 266

walking, xvi, 209–10, 214
"wearable blankets," 124, 127
weight loss
    infant, 17–21
    of mother, and breastfeeding, 84
weight monitoring, 17, 18, 20, 21
Weissbluth, Marc, *Healthy Sleep Habits,
    Happy Child*, 129–30, 172–73, 182–83,
    184, 185
wetting alarm potty training,
    245, 248

work decision, 148–58
    bottom line summary, 158
    budgeting issues, 155–57
    impacts of parental employment on child
        outcomes, 151–53
    making a choice, 157–58
    structuring the decision, 149–51
World Health Organization (WHO), 213
Wynken, Blynken, and Nod (Field), 111

Zimmerman, Frederick, 222–23